FROM THE EDITORS OF
FitPregnancy

D1378487

YOUR COMPLETE GUIDE
to a fit pregnancy

Cover photography by Pascal Demeester

Back cover photography (clockwise from top left) by Shannon Greer, Mary Ellen Bartley, David Martinez (3), Ted & Debbie

FitPregnancy

Chairman, President, CEO David Pecker
EVP, Chief Editorial Director Bonnie Fuller
EVP, Editorial Director, Active Lifestyle Group Barbara Harris

Editor In Chief Peg Moline
Art Director Stephanie Birdsong

YOUR COMPLETE GUIDE
to a fit pregnancy

Special Projects Editor Nicole Gregory
Creative Director Virginia Vincent-Orth
Editor Nancy Gottesman
Managing Editor Lily Maximo Villanueva
Fitness Editor Teri Hanson
Copy Editors Melissa Brandzel, Robin Heinz Bratslavsky, Richard Cordova
Research Editor Tajinder Rehal
Art Assistant Heather Imo
Production Director Teresa Lopas
Director Rights & Permissions Fiona Maynard
Senior Rights & Permissions Administrator Lessa Acosta
Director, Mergers & Acquisitions Jonathan J. Bigham

Contributing Writers

Kim Acosta, Connie L. Agnew, M.D., Samantha Dunn, Kim Galeaz, R.D., Jill Alison Ganon, Lu Hanessian,
Mary Jane Horton, Angela Hynes, Alice Lesch Kelly, Karen Young Kreeger, Amy Paturel, M.S., M.P.H.,
Kimberly Pfaff, Suz Redfearn, Victoria Abbott Riccardi, Shari Roan, Gayle Sato, Elizabeth Somer, M.A., R.D.,
Laura Roe Stevens, Dana Sullivan, Laurie Tarkan, Cori Vanchieri

Contributing Photographers

Henrique Bagulho, Mary Ellen Bartley, Reed Davis, Pascal Demeester, Shannon Greer, Mark Hanauer,
Lisa Hubbard, Kevin Irby, Jim Jordan, Rita Maas, David Martinez, Rob Mendolene, Victoria Pearson,
Lisa Romerein, David Roth, Ted & Debbie, David Tsay, Zee Wendell

contents

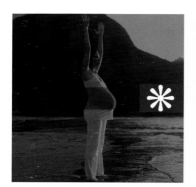

your fitness 8

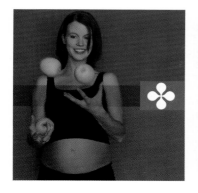

your nutrition 42

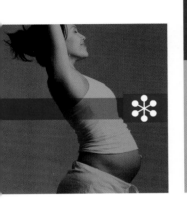

your health 70

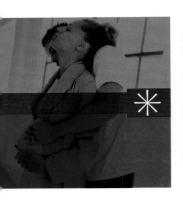

your labor and delivery 98

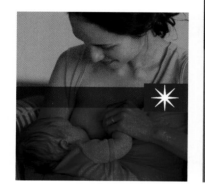

breastfeeding basics 118

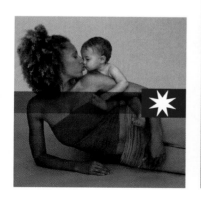

lose your baby weight 128

from the editor

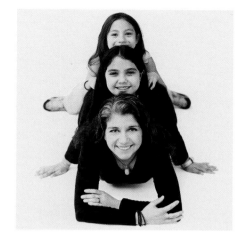

Peg with her two daughters: Lily (at age 11) and Maggie (at age 8)

expect the unexpected

> If this is your first pregnancy, you're undoubtedly bursting with questions:
- How much weight should I gain?
- Can I still work out?
- What's safe to eat?
- Why am I so _fill in your mood here_ (tired, cranky, ebullient, high-energy, low-energy—all are apt choices during these nine months)?
- What will my labor be like?
- Should I breastfeed?
- Will I ever fit into my favorite jeans again?

Well, girlfriend, you've picked up the right book. Within the pages of *Your Complete Guide to a Fit Pregnancy,* you'll find the answers to these and many more of your most-pressing questions. You'll find advice about the safest workouts for pregnant women and the wisest food choices (yes, you can eat cheddar but avoid brie and Camembert). You'll become acquainted with your body's changes—not all of which are pleasant—and your mood shifts (ditto). You'll discover what you can do now to assure successful breastfeeding (which, by the way, I strongly encourage for both your baby's and your good health). You'll get a glimpse into what to expect during delivery and the weeks beyond. Finally, with our postnatal workouts and weight-loss tips, you'll not only fit into your old jeans, you may just want to buy a new pair or two to show off your postpartum shape.

Consider this book to be your guide to becoming a mother. If you have more questions, write to me at *letterstopeg@fitpregnancy.com* and we'll try to answer your query in our bimonthly magazine.

Here's to a healthy, happy pregnancy (and new motherhood),

Peg Moline

Editor in Chief,
Fit Pregnancy magazine

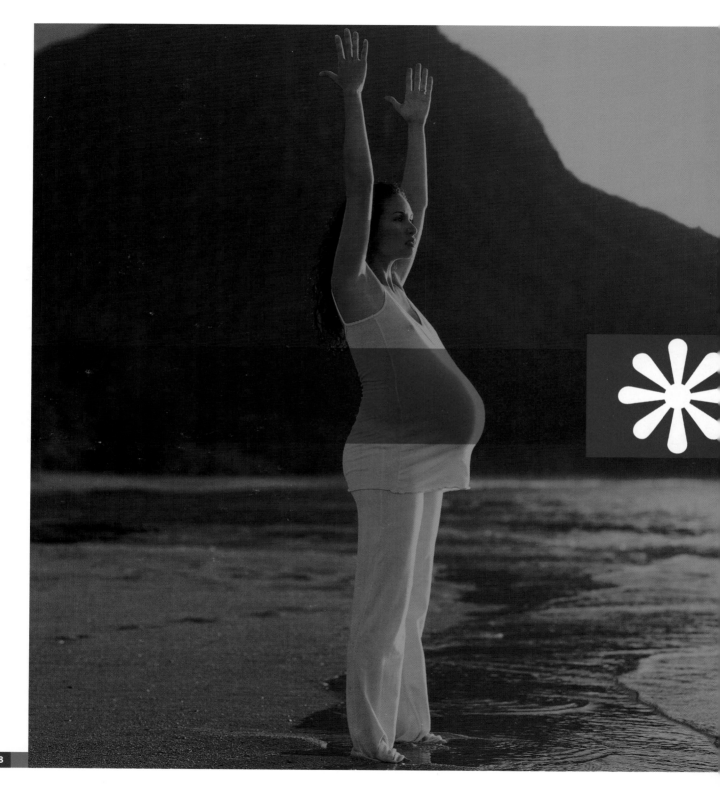

your fitness

The safest workouts for staying in shape during pregnancy

>>> WHY EXERCISE NOW, YOU ASK? Here's why: Studies have linked working out with reduced back pain, constipation and swelling as well as increased energy and better sleep. Researchers have also found that active pregnant women are less depressed and stressed than their sedentary counterparts. Although experts recommend that you engage in a variety of pleasurable physical activities, they also stress safety. The American College of Obstetricians and Gynecologists advises that all women check with their doctor before beginning any exercise program. ACOG also recommends that you avoid: 1) standing motionless for too long and exercising while lying on your back after the first trimester; 2) activities with a high risk of falling or abdominal trauma (e.g., basketball, soccer, in-line skating, downhill skiing, horseback riding, hockey, gymnastics, racquet sports); 3) scuba diving and exerting yourself at elevations higher than 6,000 feet. The workouts on these pages adhere to all of these prerequisites because we believe that pregnancy is a time to maintain your fitness, and not to push yourself too hard. Always check with your doctor before beginning any exercise program.

the safest workouts

>>> **IF YOU'VE ALWAYS EXERCISED,** you may be wondering which routines you can safely continue now that you're pregnant, and how hard you can work out. And if you haven't been active, now's the time to start moving: Research shows that exercising during pregnancy is good for you and your growing baby, and can help you get your body back in shape more quickly after you deliver.

If you wish to work with a fitness instructor, find one who is trained in prenatal exercise and can personalize your program. Here you'll find the safest, most comfortable and most effective workouts for pregnancy and information on how to get started on each of them. (For tips on when *not* to exercise, see page 33.)

walking

THE BENEFITS Walking is a great overall workout that you can do throughout your entire pregnancy to strengthen your heart and lungs while toning your lower body. Many women find that walking also boosts energy and eases nausea.

THE CAUTIONS Your joints may be more lax during pregnancy, so avoid uneven surfaces to keep from tripping and falling, particularly if your belly is large and you can't see the ground in front of you. Shorten your stride if you feel any pulling in your groin or pelvis.

HOW TO GET STARTED Walk briskly—just make sure your heel strikes first and that you roll through the arch and off the ball of your foot. Keep your abs pulled in to avoid arching your back. Try to walk at least 3–5 times a week; aim for 30 minutes each session. Monitor your intensity with the "talk test": If you can't carry on a conversation, you're working too hard.

FOR MORE INFORMATION Visit *www.fitpregnancy.com/walkingworkout*. Read *Walking Through Pregnancy and Beyond,* by Mark and Lisa Fenton and Tracy Teare (Lyons Press, 2004), which guides women of all fitness levels through pregnancy and the postpartum period. And don't miss the groundbreaking *Exercising Through Your Pregnancy,* by James F. Clapp III, M.D. (Addicus Books, 2002).

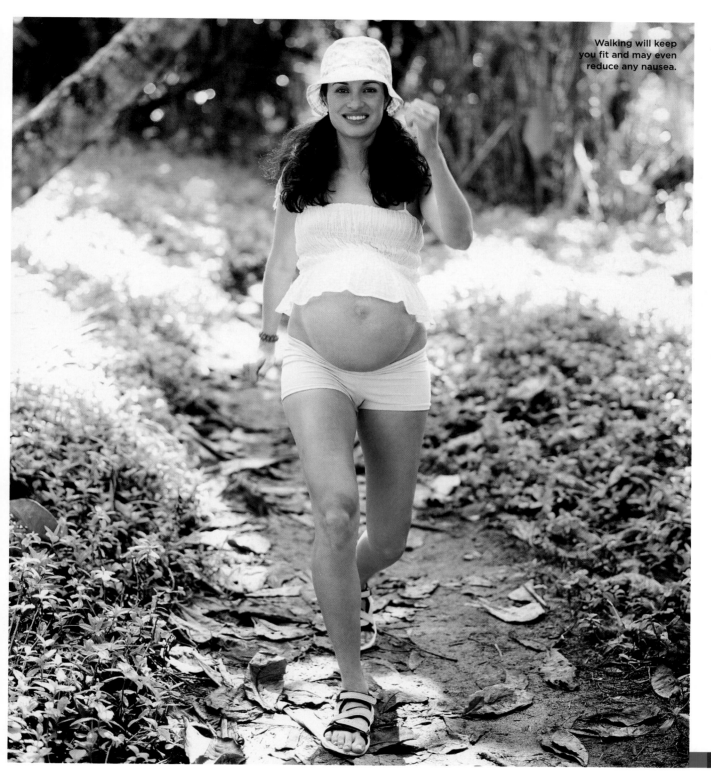

Walking will keep you fit and may even reduce any nausea.

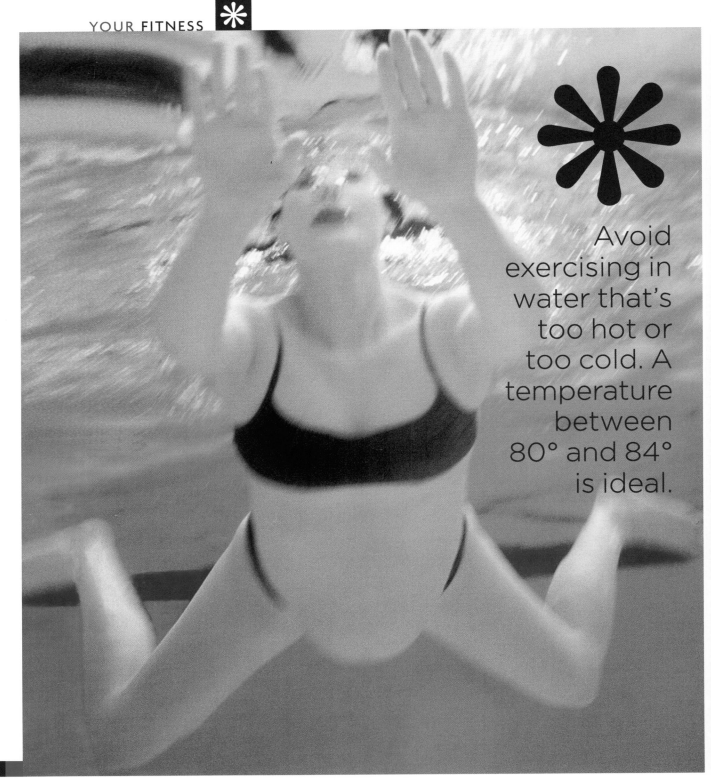

Avoid exercising in water that's too hot or too cold. A temperature between 80° and 84° is ideal.

weight training

THE BENEFITS Weight training helps maintain muscle tone, strength and proper posture. It can ease discomfort, prepare you for delivery and recovery, and help you lift and carry your baby (and all her stuff) after she arrives.

THE CAUTIONS Don't do any exercise while lying on your back after the first trimester. Reduce the amount of weight as the pregnancy progresses, and never lift your maximum weight. Maintain proper alignment and never grip the weight tightly.

HOW TO GET STARTED If you haven't previously done strength training, start slowly, using light weights. Do only 1 set of 8–12 repetitions, focusing on form. Limit training to 2–3 days a week, with a day off in between. (See page 28 for a safe, at-home strength workout.)

FOR MORE INFORMATION *Fit to Deliver,* by Karen Nordahl, M.D.; Susi Kerr; Carl Petersen, P.T., B.Sc.; and Renee Jeffreys (Hartley and Mark, 2004), is tailored to different fitness levels and stages of pregnancy. It helps women prepare for delivery and regain their prepregnancy shapes quickly during the postpartum period; visit *www.fittodeliver.com.*

water activities

THE BENEFITS Swimming, shallow-water aerobics and walking, and deep-water running offer tremendous cardiovascular benefits. The buoyancy of the water means little or no stress on your joints. Any swelling may even be reduced as the pressure of the water pushes fluids back into your bloodstream.

THE CAUTIONS Water temperature should be no warmer than 90° F. Avoid hot tubs. In addition, watch your exertion level. Keep breast or butterfly strokes to a minimum in your third trimester, as they may be too taxing on your heart. When doing shallow-water walking or pool aerobics, wear water shoes to avoid slipping.

HOW TO GET STARTED Try walking from one side of the shallow end of the pool to the other. Or hold onto the side while doing large, slow kicks and big arm circles. For a more challenging workout, use a buoyancy belt in deep water and tread water or run. If you're a swimmer, swim 20 minutes each session, 3–6 days a week. In your third trimester, swim at a lower intensity.

FOR MORE INFORMATION *Swimming Through Your Pregnancy,* by Jane Katz, D.Ed. (Doubleday, 1983), includes a safe and effective swimming and water-exercise program to keep you fit during pregnancy. It also features a 12-week postpartum program to help you get back in shape quickly.

prenatal pilates

THE BENEFITS Prenatal Pilates gently strengthens your entire body and will teach you to be aware of your pelvic-floor and transverse abdominal muscles (the deepest ab muscles), which will help you deliver your baby.

THE CAUTIONS Avoid movements that compress your neck. After the first trimester, don't work on the Reformer, which uses springs and cords that may pull too much on your hip flexors and groin muscles. During the second and third trimesters, don't attempt any inversions or do exercises lying flat on your back. Limit your range of motion as needed, and discontinue any exercise that feels uncomfortable.

HOW TO GET STARTED Use a slip-proof mat. Keep a towel nearby to relieve tension under your knees. Incorporate the Pilates breathing technique of inhaling through your nose before the movement, and exhaling through your mouth as you pull your navel to your spine and move or shift into a movement. This trains your ab and pelvic-floor muscles and will help during labor and delivery.

FOR MORE INFORMATION The *Fusion Pilates for Pregnancy* video (Gianni Productions, 2003, VHS or DVD) is designed to give women a challenging workout without compromising safety. The Pilates-based workout follows the American College of Obstetricians and Gynecologists guidelines and includes modifications appropriate for each trimester. Visit *www.fusionpilates.com*.

prenatal yoga

THE BENEFITS Prenatal yoga can be done throughout your pregnancy. The mind-body connection that you learn helps you to enjoy your changing body. You will learn how to breathe through labor pain using relaxation techniques that help your pelvic floor open up.

THE CAUTIONS Stay away from yoga classes that heat the room and classes that are too taxing. Don't attempt inverted poses such as the Headstand or Plow. Do not do any pose that requires you to lie flat on your back after the first trimester. You may want to modify such poses as Downward Dog, Triangle pose or Warrior series using a chair to help you keep your head above your heart.

HOW TO GET STARTED Since prenatal yoga programs can be very gentle, you can start one now, even if you've never set foot in a class. Become aware of your body's abilities and limitations. Listen to your breath and quiet your mind; this can be a powerful tool when it comes time to give birth. (See page 20 for a complete yoga program.)

FOR MORE INFORMATION The video *Rocki's Prenatal Yoga* (M.O.O. Productions, 2003) features a wonderful combination of standing and seated poses, breathing and relaxation techniques, and meditation that's perfect for all fitness levels. It was created by Rocki Graham, owner of Yoga Baby studio in Santa Monica, Calif. (*www.mooproductionsinc.com*).

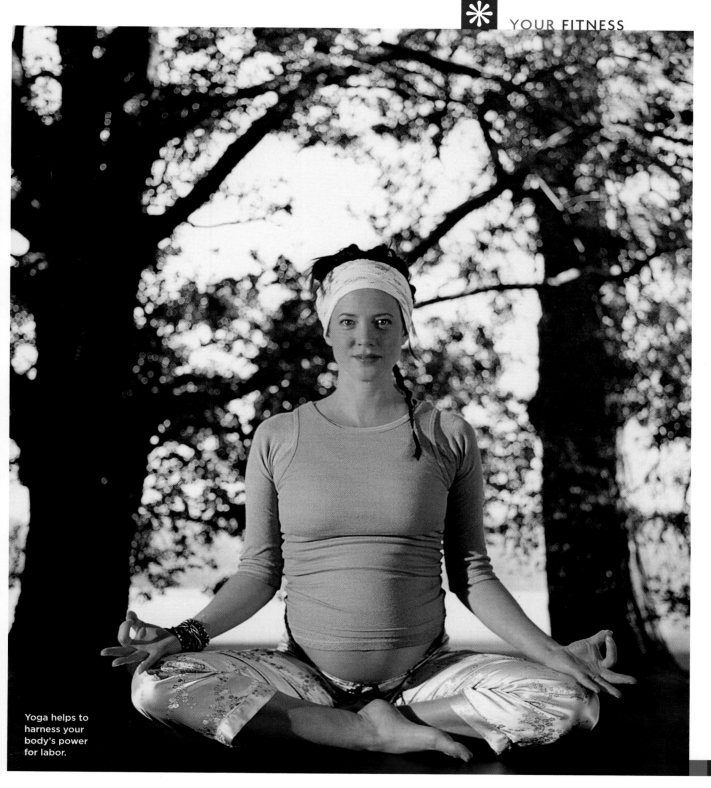

Yoga helps to
harness your
body's power
for labor.

labor prep

>>> THE PAYOFFS FOR HAVING STRONG ABDOMINAL and pelvic-floor muscles are plentiful. "These muscles are a pregnant woman's best friend," says Julie Tupler, R.N., author of *Lose Your Mummy Tummy* (Perseus, 2005) and creator of the Tupler Technique, which is illustrated in her Maternal Fitness DVD/video series (Moon Mountain Entertainment, 2001; *www.maternalfitness.com*). "If your abs are weak or if they separate from a diastasis [when the outer ab muscles separate; a condition that often occurs during pregnancy], you won't be able to push effectively," she explains. And a strong pelvic floor can help prevent urinary leaks later.

The workout on these pages, based on the Tupler Technique, teaches you to work the deep transversus abdominis, or transverse, muscle (it wraps around your torso like a girdle and involuntarily contracts when you sneeze) and the pelvic floor.

Try to do this workout up to 3 times every day. Do the exercises in the order shown, performing 10 repetitions of each move and progressing to 20 reps when you feel strong enough.

1. BELLY BREATHING

Sit on the floor with your legs crossed comfortably and your back against a support; place your hands on your belly. Without moving your back or shoulders, slowly inhale through your nose as you expand your belly. As you exhale through your mouth, draw in your abdominals, bringing your navel toward your spine (shown). *Strengthens the abdominal muscles and prepares you for the remaining exercises.*

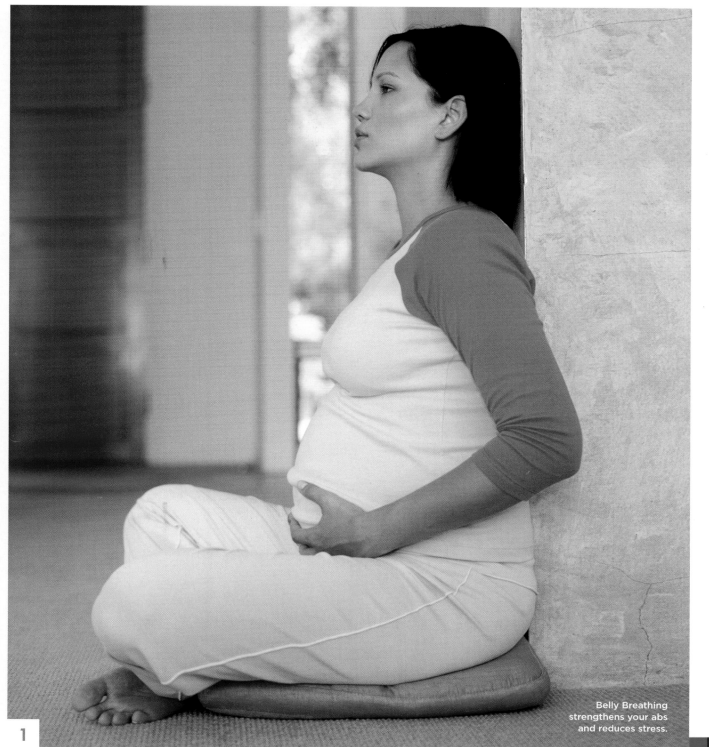

Belly Breathing strengthens your abs and reduces stress.

1

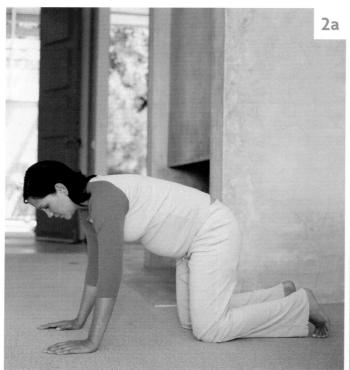

2a

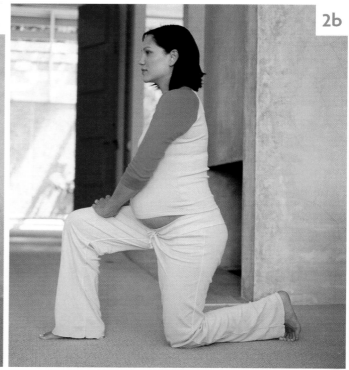

2b

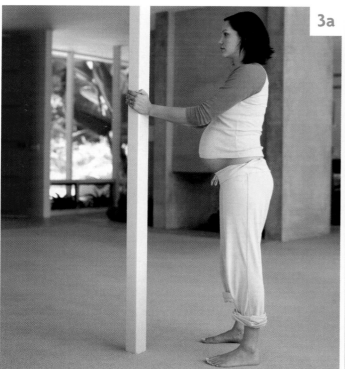

3a

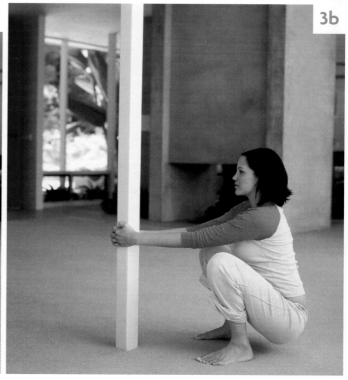

3b

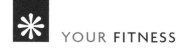
2. BELLY DANCING ON ALL FOURS

From the Belly Breathing position, kneel on all fours, knees hip-width apart, wrists under shoulders, toes curled under. With a flat back, draw the abdominals up and in by bringing the navel toward the spine and hold, breathing normally. Keeping your upper back from curving, tilt your pelvis under, bringing the pubic bone toward the navel (A). Hold and count to 5. Return to the flat-back position and repeat. When finished with the final rep, come to standing position by bringing one leg forward, foot flat on the floor, and pushing off the thigh with both hands (B). *Strengthens abdominals, back and upper body.*

3. SQUAT COMBO

Hold onto a pole for support and stand with feet wider than hip width (A). Lower into a deep squat, weight in heels (B). If heels do not touch the floor, place a towel under them. Do a Kegel and hold, counting out loud to 10. Slowly release and draw your abs in as you exhale. Remaining in squat, repeat combo 5 times, then sit down and rest. *Strengthens legs, abs and pelvic-floor muscles.*

your ab muscles & labor

THE TRANSVERSE ABDOMINIS, or transverse, is the innermost abdominal muscle and it encircles your trunk like a corset. The main muscle of the pelvic floor, the PC (short for pubo-coccygeus) lies in a figure-eight around the openings of the urethra, vagina and rectum. While pushing in labor, you ideally will work the transverse and pelvic-floor muscles separately, drawing in the transverse and relaxing the pelvic floor to let the baby out.

KEGEL EXERCISES These strengthen the pelvic-floor muscles in preparation for labor and may help prevent incontinence after you give birth. To do a Kegel (note: you don't have to be seated), squeeze the muscles around the vagina as if you are stopping the flow of urine; hold for 10 seconds, breathing normally, then slowly release. Do 20 10-second holds 5 times a day.

yoga: a simple prenatal routine

>>> THE WORD "YOGA" literally means to yoke, or join together, the body and mind. At her Golden Bridge Yoga Studio in Los Angeles, Kundalini yoga instructor Gurmukh teaches legions of pregnant women to yoke their body, breath and mind with the soul growing within them. Gurmukh has inspired expectant moms such as Madonna, Cindy Crawford and Reese Witherspoon to approach pregnancy as yoginis, or women who practice yoga.

The simple yet powerful prenatal program shown here is based on Kundalini yoga ("Kundalini" refers to the spiritual energy within the body that yoga unleashes). It was designed by Gurmukh, who is pictured with our model in some of the poses on the following pages. This routine, which can be done to your favorite music, promotes Gurmukh's message for expectant women to make the most of this special time. "Bringing a meditative element to your life now makes you more peaceful and more appreciative of the gift you have been given," she says. "It teaches you how to get in touch with your natural rhythm and energy to harness them for the stamina required during labor."

Paul Crane, M.D., an OB-GYN at Cedars-Sinai Medical Center in Los Angeles, has seen that energy in action. "Through its emphasis on concentration and breathing, yoga gives women a physical and emotional practice that can transform nicely into the birth," he says. "Their birth process often becomes an extension of their yoga practice."

For your body: Allows you to relax and focus on your breath, which helps during labor

For your mind: Allows you to appreciate the gift of your amazing pregnancy

1. miracle meditation

You can do this pose at the beginning and end of the routine. Sit in a cross-legged position with your spine straight. Bring your hands together 6 inches from your chest, pinkies touching and palms cupped. Close your eyes and remain quiet and still. Keeping your breath smooth, imagine placing everything that brings you joy in the palms of your hands. Say a silent prayer of gratitude for each of them. Rest for 3–5 breaths.

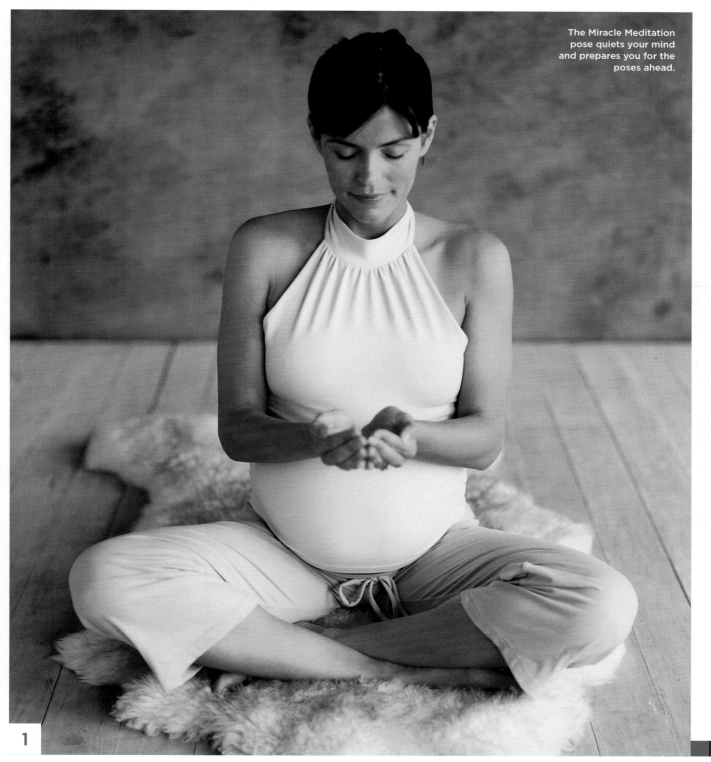

The Miracle Meditation pose quiets your mind and prepares you for the poses ahead.

1

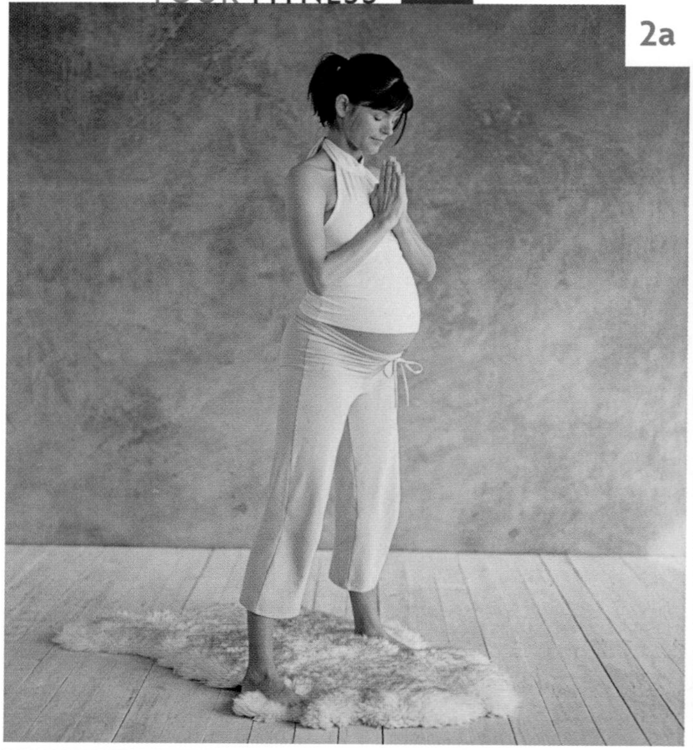

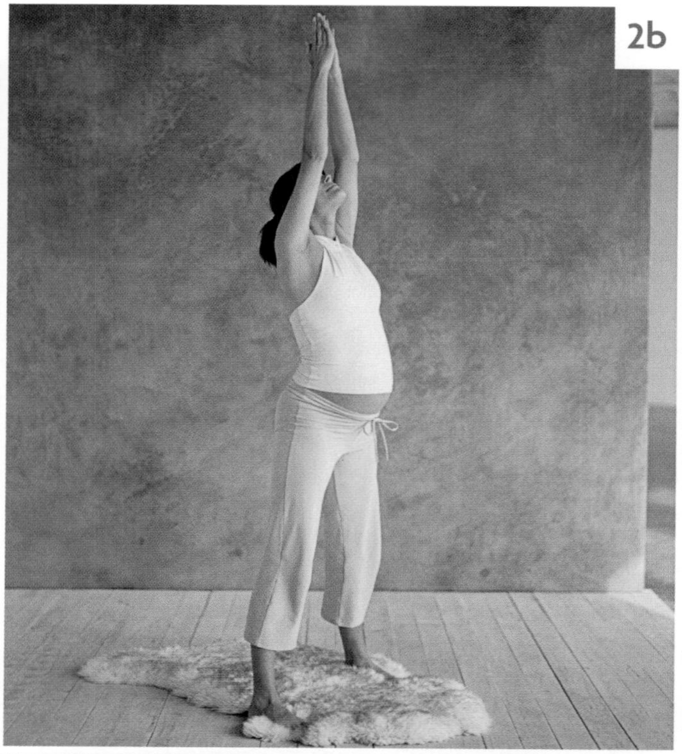

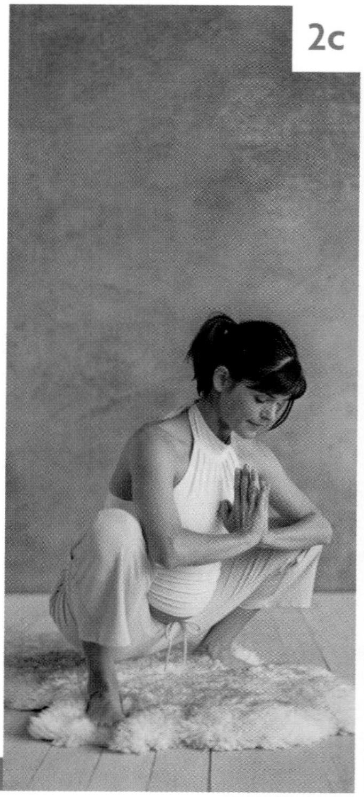

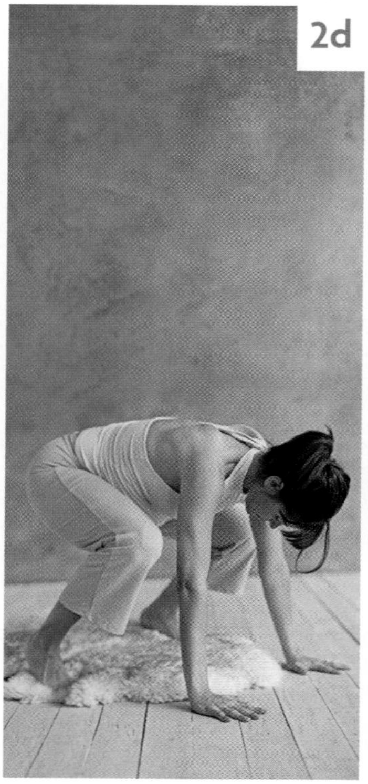

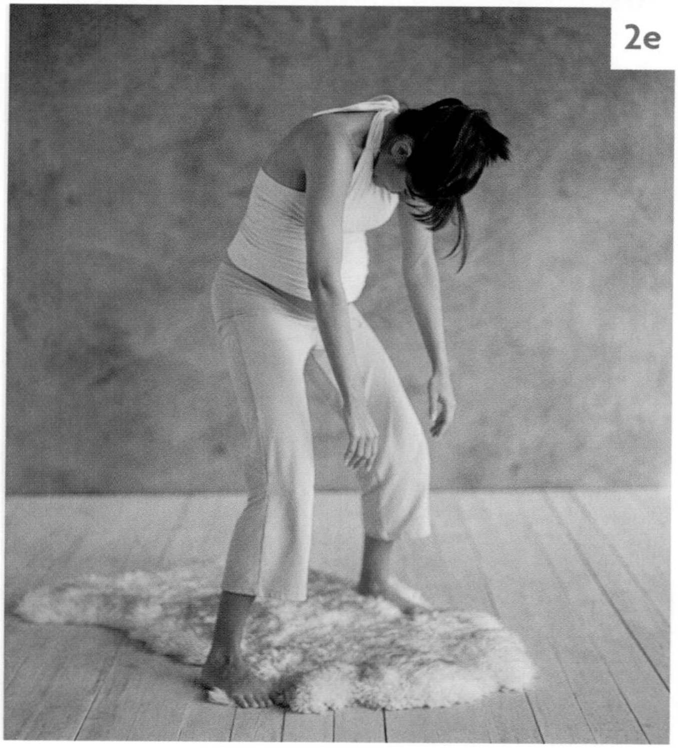

2. pregnancy yogi squat

Stand with your feet more than hip-width apart. Place hands in prayer position (A). Inhale and sweep arms out and up, keeping hands together, eyes looking up (B). Exhale as you bring your hands back to heart center and lower your body into a deep squat; hold for 1–2 breaths. Keep feet flat on the floor. (If heels come up, place a folded blanket under them.) (C) Tip forward to place hands on floor (D). Roll up to standing (E), pushing off thighs if necessary. Inhale and sweep arms out, up and back to prayer pose overhead (B). Exhale as you bring hands back to your heart center (A). Lower eyes and rest for a moment to catch your breath. Repeat for 8–10 squats, progressing to 15.

For your body: **Increases strength, stamina and flexibility**
For your mind: **Helps you feel strong; teaches you to let go and relax for labor**

3. cat cow

Get down on your hands and knees with wrists under shoulders and knees under hips, fingers spread, toes curled under, abdominals pulled up and in. Inhale through your nose and gently arc your back as you close your eyes and follow your breath (A); imagine creating space in your baby's home. Exhale through your nose and round your back, tucking chin toward chest (B). Continue this cycle for 8–10 complete breaths, progressing to 15. Sit back on heels to rest if needed.

For your body: **Stretches and strengthens abdominal and lower-back muscles**
For your mind: **Allows you to concentrate**

3a
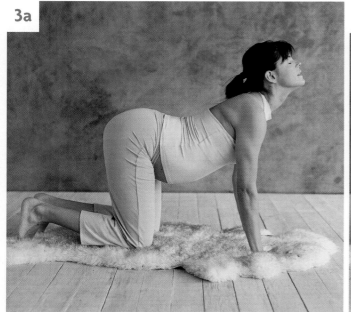

3b
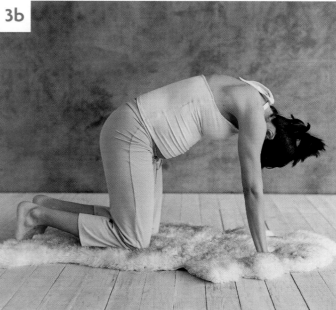

4. standing rotation

Stand with feet more than hip-width apart, knees bent. Bend forward slightly, keeping back flat, palms on thighs, fingers facing in (A). Let yourself be loose as you inhale and then exhale while you rotate your torso in an easy circular movement: up, left, down, right (B, C), giving your baby a ride. (Rotate once for each complete breath.) Continue this cycle for 8–10 breaths, progressing to 15. Repeat in opposite direction.

For your body: **Strengthens abdominal and lower-back muscles**

For your mind: **Connects with the blossoming soul growing within you**

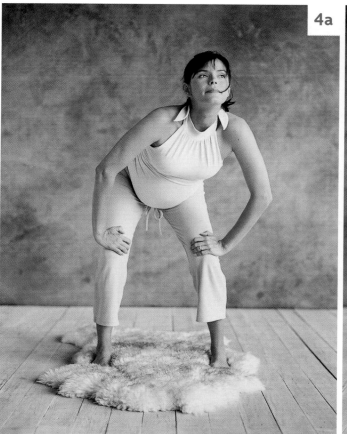

4a

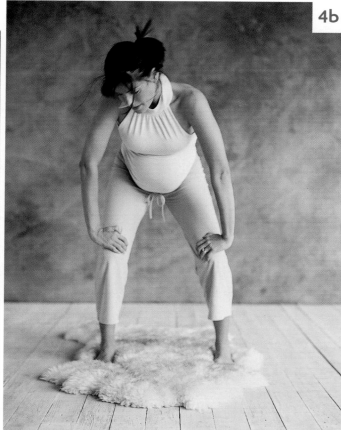

4b

As your belly grows, your center of gravity shifts forward, which can cause you to lose your balance. Yoga can help improve your stability as well as your flexibility and strength.

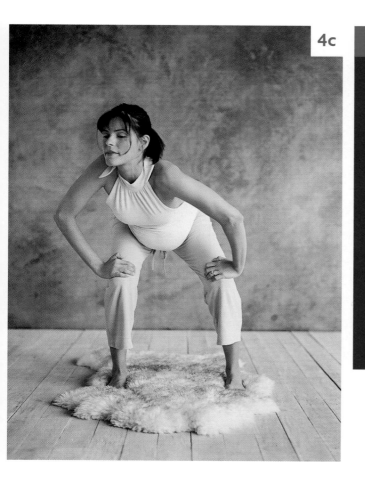

4c

practice concentration

Sit in a cross-legged position with your arms straight out to sides. Place your thumbs up with your fingers in a loose fist; close your eyes. Draw a figure eight with your thumbs, hands and arms. Breathe deeply through your nose. Continue doing this for 5–10 complete breaths, progressing to 20. This activity (not shown) teaches you to endure discomfort—such as a contraction—via breathing and concentration.

5a

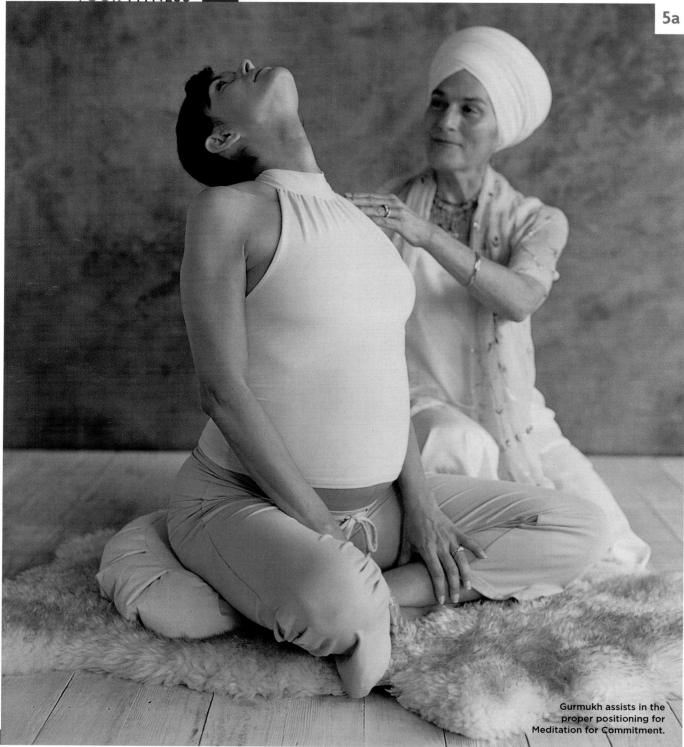

Gurmukh assists in the proper positioning for Meditation for Commitment.

5. meditation for commitment

Sit on a large pillow in a crossed-ankle position, hands resting on shins. Pull navel toward spine. Close your eyes and breathe deeply through your nose, drawing shoulder blades back and down, allowing your neck to lengthen and your head to tilt back gently. Allow your back to gently arc, opening and lifting your heart to the sky (A). Exhale through your nose and round your spine. Tuck your chin in toward your chest (B). Repeat for 8–10 full breaths, progressing to 15.

For your body: **Increases overall stamina and flexibility in the spine**
For your mind: **Makes you feel calmer and more powerful**

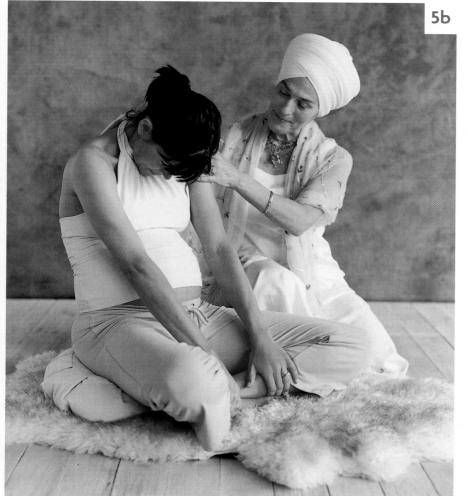

5b

good form

■ Breathe in and out through your nose, gently resting the tip of your tongue behind your teeth on the roof of your mouth.
■ Let your breath lead your movements.
■ Keep your breath smooth and slow. If your breathing becomes irregular, slow down and relax for a while.
■ Be sensitive to your body's abilities and modify the moves to suit your own energy and needs. Do not attempt any exercise that feels uncomfortable.
■ Follow your intuition. Remember, this is a practice of mental and physical conditioning. Close your eyes and go within, finding your inner strength and stamina.
■ Place a few large pillows next to you. Use one for the seated poses and have one ready for comfort as needed.

strength training: a safe at-home workout

>>> **STAYING ACTIVE DURING PREGNANCY** is one of the best things you can do for your health—and your baby's. Studies have found that pregnant women who exercise have smoother deliveries than those who aren't active and that they also feel better about themselves after delivery.

"Women who are physically fit are definitely able to handle pregnancy more easily and do the work involved in labor and delivery," says Mona Shangold, M.D., director of the Center for Women's Health and Sports Gynecology in Philadelphia. "They are also better able to handle the physical demands after delivery: carrying a baby and all of the paraphernalia involved."

Weight training, in particular, helps prepare you for the hard work of labor and new motherhood. Our at-home strength-training program, with options for working out at the gym, is just the ticket to help you maintain your muscle tone and current level of fitness. In addition to this workout, try to participate in an aerobic activity of your choice at least 3 times per week for a minimum of 20 minutes each time.

As with any exercise during pregnancy, it's best to talk to your doctor before beginning our workout routine, Shangold says. (For tips on when *not* to exercise, see "Caution!" on page 33.)

good form

■ Always begin your workouts with a 5-minute warm-up such as walking or shoulder, neck and ankle rolls. End with a 5-minute cool-down that stretches every muscle worked.

■ Keep your abs contracted, navel pulled toward spine and tailbone pointing down.

■ Keep your neck relaxed when pulling your shoulder blades back and down.

■ Most standing exercises, unless otherwise noted, should be done with feet wider than hip-width apart; use a wider stance if needed to accommodate your growing belly.

■ Use slow, controlled movements to protect your joints, which tend to become loose during pregnancy.

■ Breathe! Inhale through your nose before you go into the move and exhale as you execute the move. Don't hold your breath.

■ Don't grip weights too tightly; this can cause blood pressure to rise.

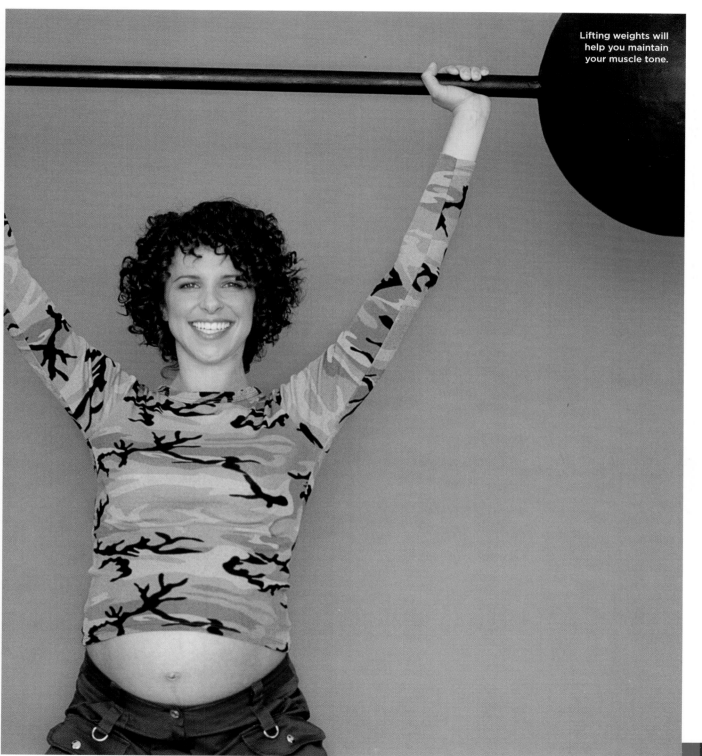

Lifting weights will help you maintain your muscle tone.

the workout

If you were strength training regularly prior to becoming pregnant, do 1–2 sets of 8–15 reps for each move of this workout about 2–3 times a week. Otherwise, start with just 1–2 sets of 8–10 reps twice a week.

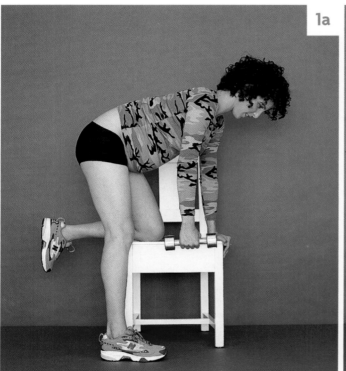

1a

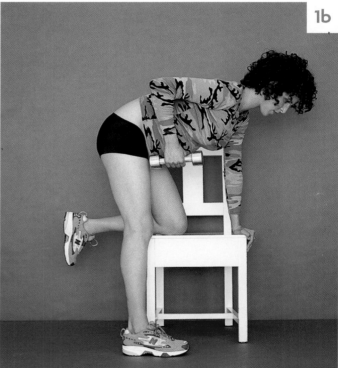

1b

1. one-arm row

Place your left hand and left knee on the seat of a chair. Lean forward, holding a dumbbell in your right hand; keep right arm straight, palm facing in (A). Bend right elbow, pulling dumbbell toward waist, and pause (B). Return to starting position and repeat for reps; switch legs and repeat with other arm. Recommended weight: 5–8 pounds.

Gym option: Use one cable of the seated cable row machine. *Strengthens middle back and biceps.*

Toning your upper and lower body is a great way to stay strong for childbirth—and whatever your new life as a mom has in store for you.

2. curl and lift

Sit on the edge of a chair with your knees bent, feet flat on floor. Hold a dumbbell in each hand, arms straight and by your sides, palms facing in. Bend elbows, raising forearms parallel to floor (A). Lift arms up to shoulder height, keeping elbows bent, upper arms parallel to floor (B). Lower arms back to sides, then return to starting position; repeat for reps. Recommended weight: 5–8 pounds.

Gym option: Same as above. *Strengthens biceps and shoulders.*

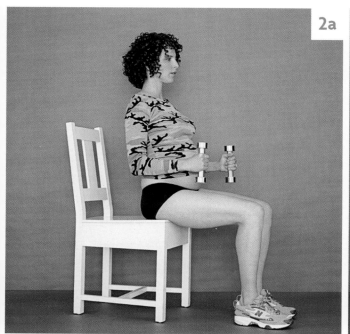

2a

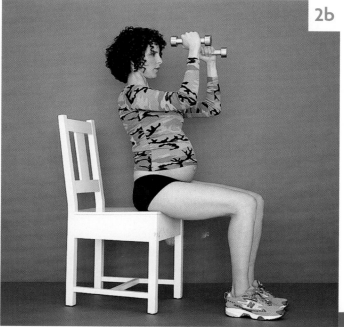

2b

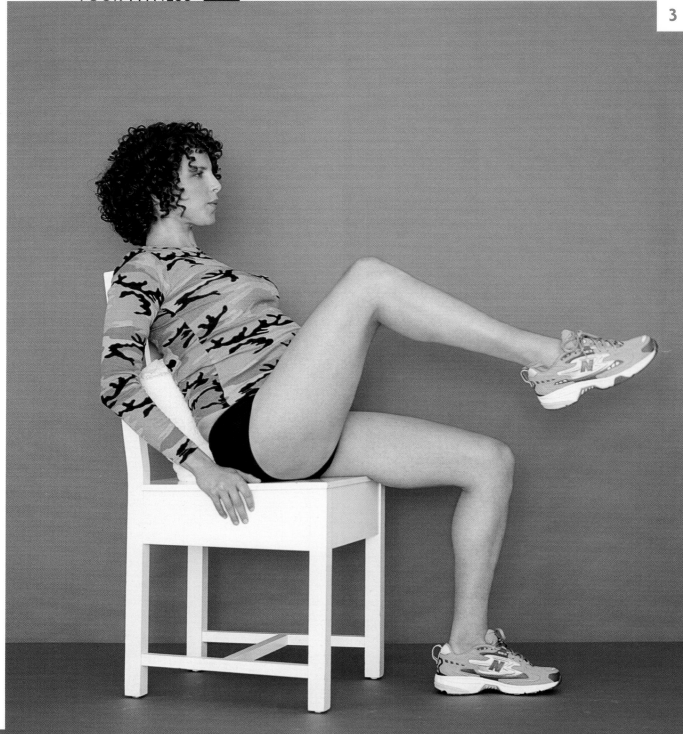

3. seated ab

Sit on the edge of a chair with your knees bent and your feet flat on the floor. Keeping your abs tight, lean back so only your upper back and shoulders are supported by the chair back. (Prop a pillow behind you if necessary.) Inhale and hold, then exhale and bend your right knee up toward chest (shown). Lower foot to floor, then alternate with other leg. Repeat for reps.

Gym option: Same exercise described above using an incline bench. *Strengthens abdominals.*

4. chest fly

Sit on the chair with a pillow propped behind you. Bend your knees and place feet flat on floor. Holding a dumbbell in each hand, extend arms directly above your chest, elbows slightly bent, knuckles touching (A). Inhale; open arms out just to the point of a mild stretch without arching your back (B). Exhale and press arms together; repeat for reps. Recommended weight: 5–12 pounds.

Gym option: Use the chest fly machine. *Strengthens chest, front shoulders and triceps.*

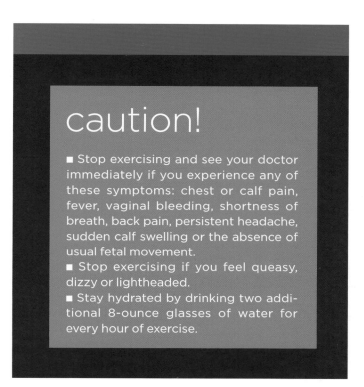

caution!

■ Stop exercising and see your doctor immediately if you experience any of these symptoms: chest or calf pain, fever, vaginal bleeding, shortness of breath, back pain, persistent headache, sudden calf swelling or the absence of usual fetal movement.
■ Stop exercising if you feel queasy, dizzy or lightheaded.
■ Stay hydrated by drinking two additional 8-ounce glasses of water for every hour of exercise.

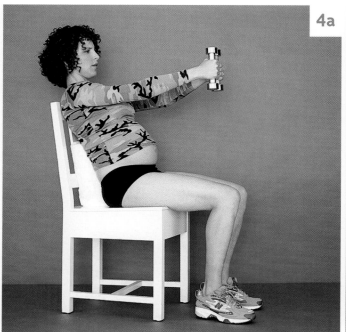

4a

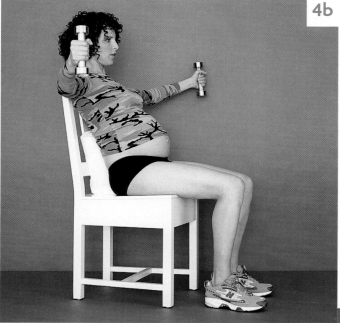

4b

Lower-body strength is important for carrying the added weight of pregnancy efficiently and gracefully.

5. plié

Stand with your left side to the back of a chair and your toes and knees turned out about 45 degrees, left hand on chair for support and right elbow bent at an angle, right hand on hip. Bend knees, lowering torso as much as possible without shifting pelvis (shown). Press into your heels as you straighten legs to return to starting position; repeat for reps.

Gym option: Same exercise, holding onto back of incline bench. *Strengthens quadriceps, hamstrings and buttocks.*

6. standing hamstring curl

Attach an ankle weight to your right ankle and stand facing the back of a chair with feet slightly separated. Bring right foot slightly behind you, toes touching the floor, knee bent (A). Bend your right knee upward and flex foot to bring right heel toward buttocks (B). Return to starting position and repeat for reps, then switch ankle weight to other leg and repeat. Recommended weight: 2–4 pounds.

Gym option: Use a seated or standing hamstring curl machine. *Strengthens hamstrings.*

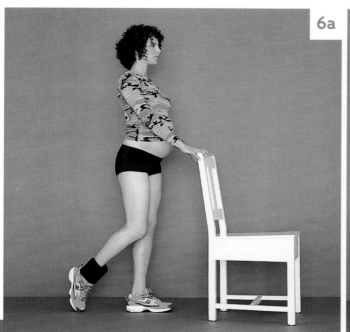

6a

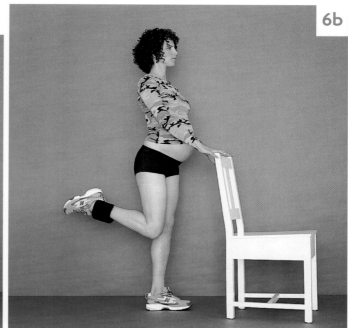

6b

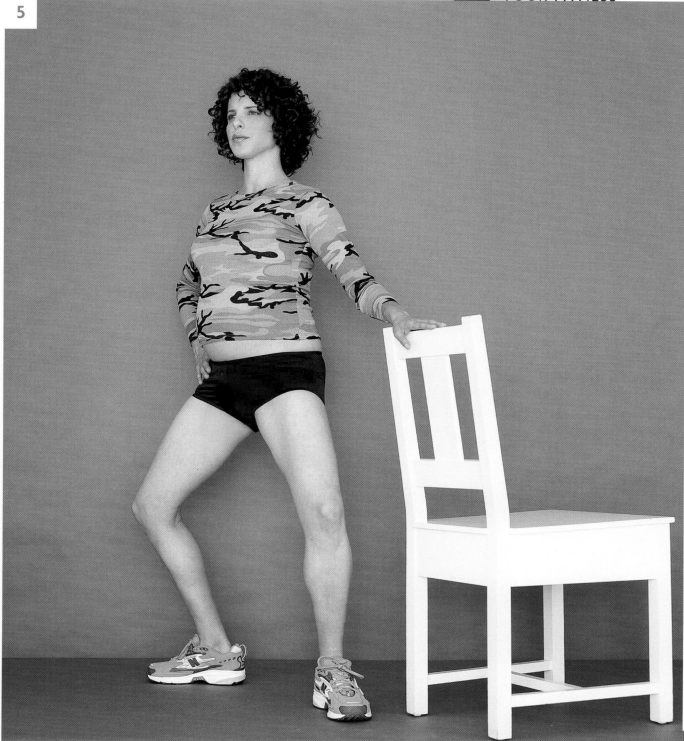

fitness remedies

>>> **NO QUESTION ABOUT IT: Working out agrees with pregnant women. Cardiovascular workouts (like walking, swimming and running) boost your energy and stamina. Weight lifting improves your strength. And yoga helps you feel balanced—both mentally and physically—as well as serene and more flexible. All of this will help you during your labor and delivery—and beyond. But exercise has yet another function for the expectant mother: Certain types of physical activity can banish pregnancy aches and pains. Here, four fitness solutions to some common pregnancy problems.**

1.
THE PROBLEM>FEELING HEAVY
THE SOLUTION>SWIMMING

Why it works > In bodies of water, a pregnant woman feels weightless; the water's buoyancy lifts the burden of gravity and helps shrink swelling. "The pressure of the water against your skin forces much of the extra fluid—usually gathering in your legs and feet—back into the bloodstream," says Cincinnati physical therapist Gail Wehrman, who specializes in women's health. From there, the excess fluid heads to the kidneys, you urinate it out and, thus, the swelling goes down. "But to get the most of this effect, you must dwell in the deeper end of the pool," Wehrman says, "where the water can press against every part of your body that is swelling." And you must move around. Try deep-water aerobics, water Pilates or the bikes that some gyms now offer in pools.

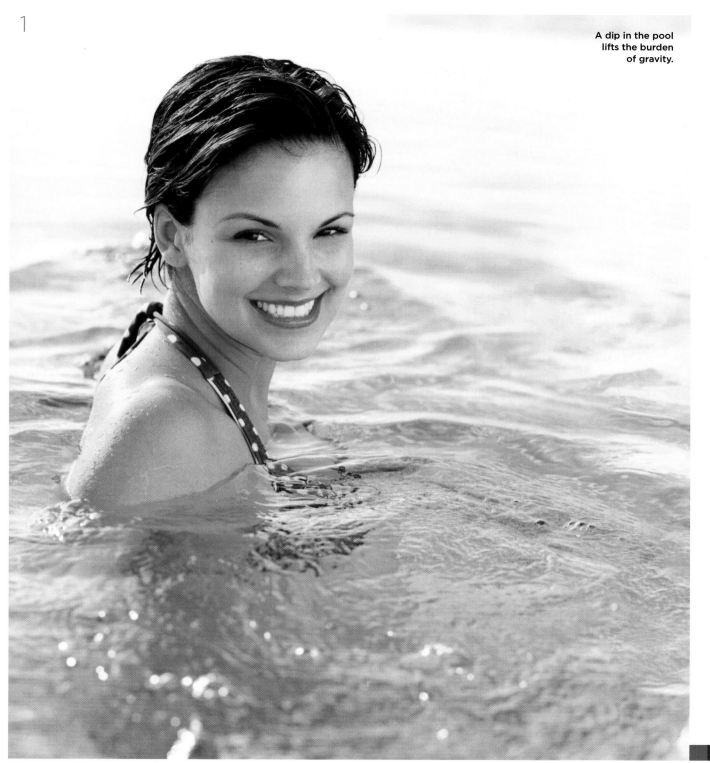

A dip in the pool
lifts the burden
of gravity.

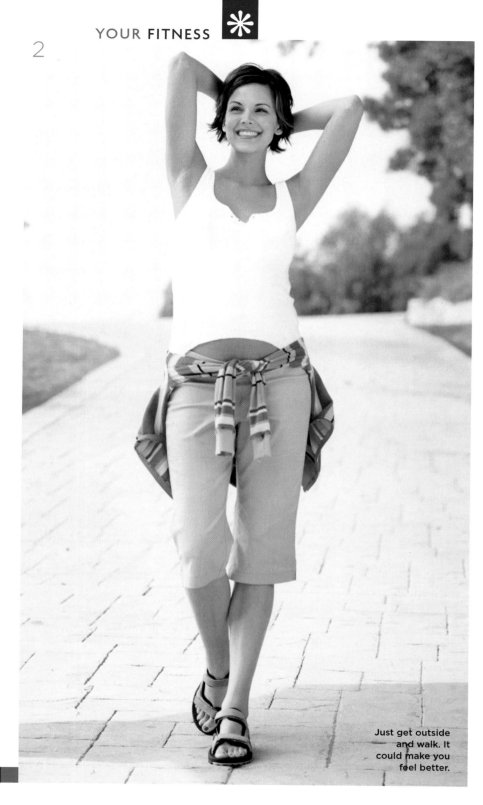

Just get outside and walk. It could make you feel better.

2.
THE PROBLEM>NAUSEA
THE SOLUTION>WALKING

Why it works > Scientists aren't sure why walking alleviates nausea—they just know it does, says exercise physiologist and prenatal fitness expert Renee Jeffreys of Covington, Ky. It could be that a moderate walk shunts blood away from the midriff and out to the limbs, where it's needed for movement. Whether you're up for a long, short, fast or slow walk, just get outside— or on the treadmill—for five or 10 minutes and see how it feels. If you feel better, continue for 30 minutes more. If your nausea worsens or if you experience other symptoms, call your doctor.

4.
THE PROBLEM>RADIATING UPPER-THIGH PAIN
THE SOLUTION>STANDING HIP-FLEXOR STRETCH

Why it works > Pain that radiates through the upper thighs and sometimes down the calves is often the result of hip dysfunction ushered in by the pregnancy hormone relaxin, which loosens and widens the hip joint in preparation for childbirth. The hip-flexor stretch (see opposite page) can relieve tension and help move loosened muscles back into alignment. But if you're suffering from calf cramps of the charley-horse variety, you could be deficient in potassium or calcium. Talk with your doctor about your diet and/or supplements; in the meantime, try sitting in a chair and flexing your toes upward to relieve pain.

3.

THE PROBLEM>CARPAL TUNNEL SYNDROME
THE SOLUTION>ARM ELEVATION, FIVE-
FINGER STRETCH

Why it works > As early as the first six weeks of pregnancy, swelling in the tissues of the hand and wrist can increase, pinching the median nerve, which brings feeling to many of your fingers. The numbness, tingling and pain that follow can be relieved by elevating your hands above your heart and gently extending your fingers (shown at right), says Robert M. Szabo, M.D., M.P.H., a surgeon and professor of orthopedic surgery at the University of California, Davis, School of Medicine. This pumps fluid out of the swollen tissues that surround the nerve. But whatever you do, don't try to exercise your wrist by bending it to extremes, as this will only cause more pain and possibly injury. Experts also suggest wearing a loose splint at night to minimize movement, thus preventing pressure on the nerve. If possible, avoid tasks that require forceful, repetitive hand movements; such actions can aggravate your symptoms.

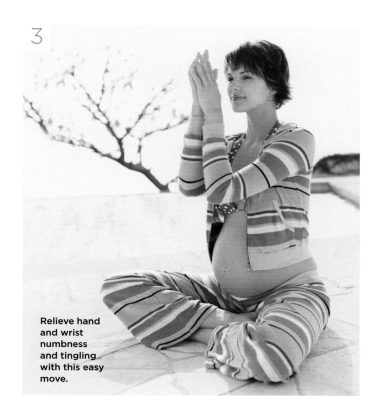

3

Relieve hand and wrist numbness and tingling with this easy move.

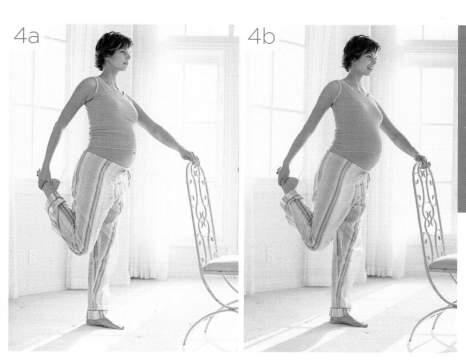

4a

4b

The move > Stand with your feet hip-width apart, holding the back of a chair or couch. Bend your right knee to bring heel toward your buttocks. Hold your right foot, knees together, buttocks contracted (A). Tilt pelvis down and pull right leg back until you feel a mild stretch in your upper right thigh (B). Hold for at least 30 seconds, then switch sides. Repeat as needed.

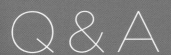

>>> ANSWERS to your questions about the best (read: safest) exercises to perform during your pregnancy.

Q I'm very close to the end of my first trimester. Why can't I continue to do exercises that require me to lie on my back?

A The weight of your uterus increases throughout pregnancy, so if you were to spend time lying flat on your back, that extra weight might compress the vena cava, the large blood vessel that runs along your spine and carries blood to the heart. Compression of this vein may cause you to become dizzy, lightheaded, nauseated or sweaty, and it may briefly reduce blood flow to your baby. For this reason, you should avoid the supine, or flat-on-the-back, position after about the third month (though some supine exercises can be modified by doing them on your side or by propping up your back and shoulders with pillows). You should also speak with your doctor to be sure you are following safe practices while exercising.

Q I'm 28 weeks pregnant and love to exercise, but I've just been placed on bed rest because of premature labor. Are there any exercises that I can safely do while in bed?

A Yes, you can work with your doctor and a physical therapist to develop a gentle exercise plan. Keep in mind, however, that this is not the time for aerobic workouts or muscle strengthening. The goal of exercise while on bed rest is to minimize the risk of developing blood clots in your extremities.

Physical therapist Cam Lippincott, director of rehabilitation medicine at Glendale Memorial Hospital in Glendale, Calif., suggests that women on bed rest do range-of-motion exercises (moving each joint as far as it can go in every direction) for their ankles, knees, wrists, elbows and shoulders.

You might also visit *www.sidelines.org*, which provides support to expectant mothers on bed rest.

Q I am in my first trimester and recently read that pregnant women should not exercise at altitudes higher than 6,000 feet. I live at 5,300 feet and frequently hike at 8,000 feet. Should I stop?

A There is evidence that exercise at elevations higher than 6,000 feet may cause changes in heart rate, lung capacity and other cardiopulmonary measures that could cause complications. But this does not necessarily apply to women who are used to exercising at higher elevations. Your hikes probably are fine (but do check with your doctor). Still, modify the intensity in your second and third trimesters. Be aware of overexertion; symptoms include uterine contractions, excessive perspiration and increased shortness of breath.

Q I've been doing Pilates for almost a year, and I'd like to continue if possible. What are your thoughts about such exercise during pregnancy?

A Pilates is a wonderful activity that you can continue throughout pregnancy with some modification. It offers gentle muscle strengthening while improving balance, which can be a real benefit as your body's shape evolves.

Pilates is often done on an apparatus with spring-resistant bars, but getting on and off during the second and third trimesters can be awkward and pose a risk of falling. We recommend that Pilates workouts be done exclusively on floor mats once the second trimester begins. As you probably know, you should not work out lying flat on your back in your second and third trimesters. Instead, use a hip wedge, raise your upper torso or do exercises on your side.

While some Pilates studios offer their own instructor-certification programs, there is currently no national licensing procedure. You should therefore make sure that you are working with an instructor who is knowledgeable about exercising safely during pregnancy.

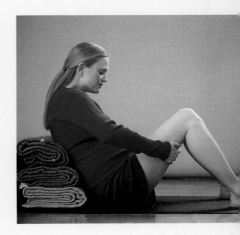

Q I'm 28 years old and in my last trimester. I swim almost every day, but my aunt says I should stop soon because if my water breaks in the pool, I might not be aware of it and it could be a problem. Is this true?

A While your aunt undoubtedly is thinking only of your best interests, swimming daily is a real gift to you and your unborn baby that poses no danger even as you approach your due date. If your water breaks while you are in the pool—or the bathtub, for that matter—you will feel the fluid leaking and should contact your doctor immediately. The real concern is that you take every precaution to steady yourself getting into and out of the pool or tub. The hazards of losing your footing on slippery tile are greater than the likelihood of any complications resulting from your water breaking while you swim.

Q I'm an aerobics instructor in my fifth month of pregnancy. Can I continue doing abdominal exercises until the baby is born?

A As mentioned earlier, the main concern about abdominal exercise is that lying on your back can cause the increased weight of your uterus to compress the vena cava vein, which carries blood to the heart. To be safe, do your ab exercises sitting in a chair or on the floor with a support behind your lower back. Inhale through your nose and expand your belly. As you exhale through your mouth, draw your navel in toward your spine. Prop up your back and shoulders with pillows. For an excellent DVD/video series featuring prenatal abdominal exercises, visit *www.maternalfitness.com.*

Q I've been a Spinning enthusiast for several years. Is it OK to continue now that I'm pregnant?

A The concern about Spinning—a supercharged, indoor stationary cycling workout—during pregnancy is that it usually causes significant dehydration and a very high heart rate. We therefore take a cautious approach and suggest that you stop the program while pregnant. Less-intense aerobic exercises, such as brisk walking or swimming, are safer but still rigorous enough to give you the desired health benefits.

   If you still want to continue Spinning, discuss this possibility with your doctor. If she gives you the go-ahead to continue, resist the temptation to spin more vigorously than you should: Use the "talk test" and do not spin to the point where your speech and breathing are labored. Also, keep water next to your bike and drink it throughout the workout so you don't become dehydrated.

Q I'm 19 weeks pregnant and an expert in-line skater. Can I safely continue skating throughout my pregnancy?

A No. There is the possibility of trauma to your unprotected abdomen should you fall, and at 19 weeks, such a trauma could put your pregnancy at risk. As is the case for all balance-related athletic activities, unexpected circumstances such as someone running out in front of you, or unanticipated conditions such as a bump or crack in the sidewalk, can cause even you, an expert in-line skater, to fall. Walking, power-walking, stationary cycling or swimming are excellent fitness alternatives for now.

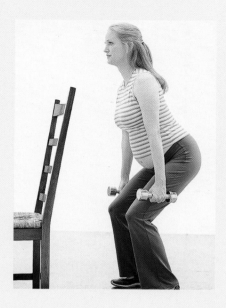

Q I'm six weeks pregnant and have been lifting weights for three years. I weigh 120 pounds and squat 90 pounds—can I continue using heavy weights while doing semisquats?

A No. A semisquat that has you rising with 90 pounds borne across your shoulders is not an exercise you should be doing during pregnancy—it exerts too much pressure on your back, knees and pelvic-floor muscles. A deep squat *without* weights is the best move you can do to strengthen your legs, hips, buttocks and abdominals (see page 22 to learn how to do a deep squat properly).

   Pregnant women who are weight lifting with machines should switch to dumbbells and reduce the weight by at least 50 percent, as multiple repetitions of light weights are safer than fewer reps with heavier weights. And a pregnant woman who has never used free weights should use 2- to 5-pound dumbbells.

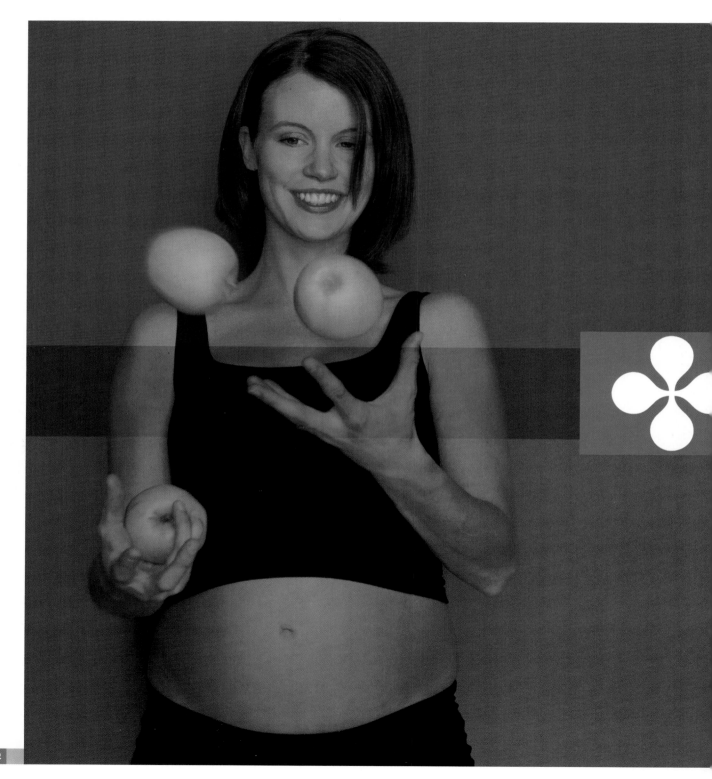

your
nutrition

>>> YOU PROBABLY ALREADY KNOW that for the next nine months (longer if you breastfeed), your growing baby is dependent on you for all the nutrients she needs. What you may not know is that your current diet can affect your baby for her entire life. Indeed, some health conditions, such as cancer and diabetes, have been linked to poor prenatal nutrition. Inadequate intake of one or more essential nutrients during critical periods in an organ's growth also can permanently alter the size of that organ. Furthermore, researchers suspect that poor nutrition during fetal development increases a child's lifelong risk for heart disease, high blood pressure and impaired glucose tolerance. But getting adequate nutrition for you and your baby doesn't mean you have to become obsessed about every morsel. In the pages of this chapter, you'll find all the nutritional information you need for the next nine months—and beyond!

in this chapter:
- ❖ a diet for the future: your three-trimester meal plan (+ recipes)
- ❖ how much weight should you gain?
- ❖ the do's and dont's of your prenatal diet
- ❖ the fab 5
- ❖ what's safe to eat, what's not
- ❖ the truth about baby weight
- ❖ Q & A

a diet for the future

>>> ALTHOUGH IT TAKES ABOUT 56,000 extra calories to make a healthy baby, that equates to only 300 extra calories a day (the equivalent of a glass of low-fat milk, a slice of bread and an apple). And that's only in the last two trimesters. Calorie needs during the first trimester are about 2,000 to 2,200 a day, the same as for nonpregnant women.

Your vitamin and mineral needs skyrocket during pregnancy, however. You need more vitamin A, folate and iron, as well as increased amounts of most other nutrients. That means you need to consume a lot more fruits, vegetables, whole grains, legumes and milk.

Your responsibility is great, but you needn't be overwhelmed. Focus on a variety of minimally processed, nutrient-dense foods and you can rest assured you're providing your baby with everything she needs for healthy growth and development. Our mix-and-match three-trimester meal plan below will help you choose the right foods to do just that.

your 3-trimester meal plan

During all three trimesters, choose one item from each category for each meal, plus an additional choice from the vegetables category at dinner (on page 49). Also choose three items from the snacks section (page 47) throughout the day. During your second and third trimesters, add an item from the second-and-third-trimesters category at lunch and dinner. If you're counting: First-trimester menus equal about 2,200 calories per day; second- and third-trimester menus equal about 2,500 calories per day.

breakfast

grains (pick 1)

$^2/_3$ cup oatmeal cooked in $^2/_3$ cup low-fat (2%) milk, topped with 2 tablespoons raisins, 1 tablespoon chopped walnuts and 1 tablespoon brown sugar

1 whole-wheat English muffin, toasted and topped with 2 tablespoons peanut or soy-nut butter

1 cup shredded-wheat cereal topped with 1 tablespoon chopped almonds, 2 tablespoons dried cranberries and 1 rounded tablespoon brown sugar

2 whole-grain frozen waffles, toasted and topped with 2 tablespoons berry or maple syrup

1 3-ounce bran muffin with 2 tablespoons peanut butter or cashew-nut butter

2 slices French toast (made with 1 large egg, 2 tablespoons low-fat milk, 1 tablespoon sugar and 1 teaspoon vanilla extract)

calcium (pick 1)

1 cup vanilla soy milk, fortified with calcium and vitamin D

1 cup low-fat (2%) milk

6 ounces low-fat yogurt

1 ounce cheddar cheese

Hot cocoa (made with $^1/_2$ cup low-fat milk, $^1/_2$ cup water and 1 packet sugar-free cocoa mix)

fruits (pick 1)

1 large navel orange

$^1/_2$ cup stewed prunes

1 $^1/_4$ cup blueberries

2 cups cantaloupe or honeydew melon, cubed

2 $^1/_2$ cups strawberries

1 banana (dust with cinnamon powder if desired)

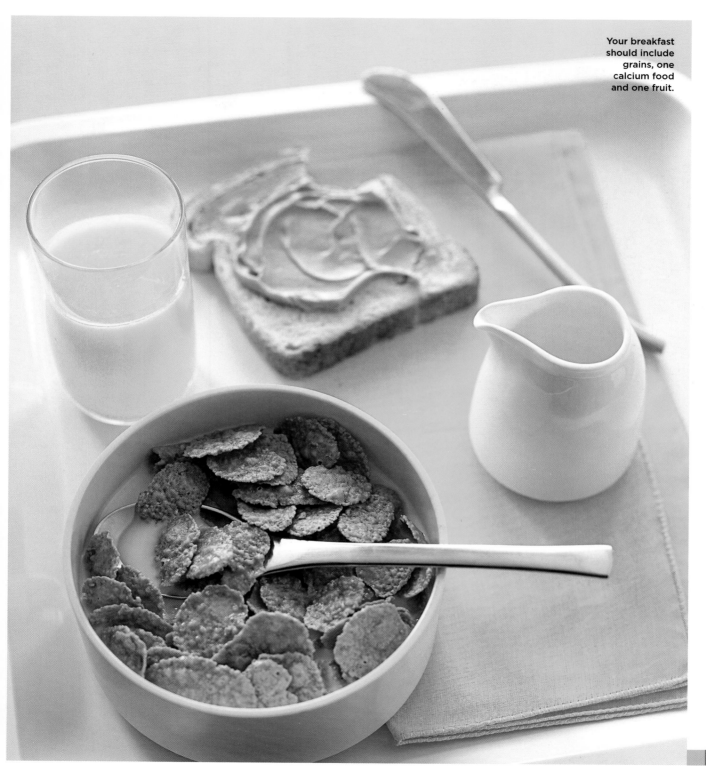

Your breakfast should include grains, one calcium food and one fruit.

What you eat during the next nine months of your pregnancy can set the stage for your child's lifelong health.

lunch

entree (pick 1)

Turkey sandwich: 2 ounces turkey meat, 2 slices whole-wheat bread, 2 tablespoons cranberry sauce, 1 lettuce leaf and 2 teaspoons mayonnaise.

Grilled vegetable sandwich: 2 slices eggplant and $1/3$ red pepper, cut into slices, brushed with 1 teaspoon olive oil and grilled in a skillet. Place on 2 slices of French bread with 1 slice low-fat mozzarella cheese. Drizzle with $1/2$ teaspoon balsamic vinegar.

1 cup split-pea soup with 1 small piece of cornbread

Grilled-chicken Caesar salad: 2 cups romaine lettuce topped with 1 medium tomato, chopped; 3 ounces grilled chicken breast; and 5 teaspoons Caesar salad dressing.

1 whole-wheat pita bread, torn into pieces and dipped in $1/2$ cup hummus

Beef and bean burrito: 1 10-inch flour tortilla filled with 2 ounces extra-lean cooked beef; $1/4$ cup refried beans; 1 medium tomato, chopped; 3 tablespoons corn kernels; and 2 tablespoons salsa.

calcium (pick 1)

1 cup vanilla soy milk, fortified with calcium and vitamin D

1 cup low-fat (2%) milk

6 ounces low-fat fruit-flavored yogurt

1 ounce Monterey Jack cheese

$2/3$ cup low-fat milk, warmed, flavored with vanilla and nutmeg

fruits & vegetables (pick 1)

$2^1/_2$ cups papaya

Carrot-raisin salad: $1/2$ cup grated carrots, 2 teaspoons raisins, 1 teaspoon lemon juice, 1 teaspoon sugar, 2 teaspoons mayonnaise.

Spinach-pear salad: 1 cup fresh spinach leaves; $1/2$ pear, sliced; 4 cucumber slices; 1 tablespoon bean sprouts; and 2 teaspoons French dressing.

Vegetable platter: 1 cup broccoli florets, 10 baby carrots, $1/4$ cup sliced jicama and 3 mushrooms. Serve with 4 teaspoons sour-cream-and-onion dip.

Fruit salad: 1 kiwi, peeled and sliced; $1/2$ small can mandarin oranges, drained; $1/2$ banana, sliced; 10 fresh raspberries; and $1/2$ teaspoon candied ginger, crumbled.

Three-bean salad: $1/4$ cup cooked kidney beans, $1/4$ cup cooked green beans, $1/4$ cup cooked garbanzo beans and 3 tablespoons thinly sliced red onion, tossed with 2 tablespoons balsamic vinegar, 2 teaspoons olive oil and $1/2$ teaspoon fresh dill.

in 2nd & 3rd trimesters (pick 1)

1 large orange

1 medium apple, cored and sprinkled with cinnamon

1 steamed artichoke with yogurt dip (2 tablespoons low-fat yogurt mixed with lemon juice and pepper to taste)

5 vanilla wafers

$1/2$ cup fruit sorbet

snacks

(pick 3 a day)

- 1 mango
- 4 cups air-popped popcorn
- 2 cups strawberries drizzled with 1 tablespoon chocolate syrup
- 2 graham crackers topped with 2 teaspoons peanut butter
- Celery sticks topped with 1 tablespoon peanut butter
- 1½ cups frozen blueberries
- Cranberry spritzer: Mix 8 ounces cranberry juice with 8 ounces sparkling water, ice cubes and a twist of lemon.
- 1 large baked apple
- 1 slice cinnamon-raisin bread dipped in 4 tablespoons low-fat cinnamon-apple yogurt
- ⅔ cup pineapple chunks with ⅓ cup cottage cheese

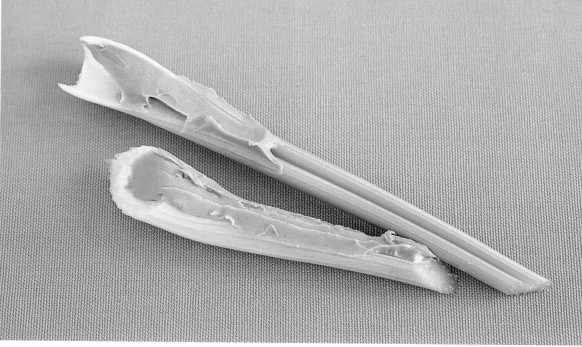

Snacking at regular intervals will keep your energy level up.

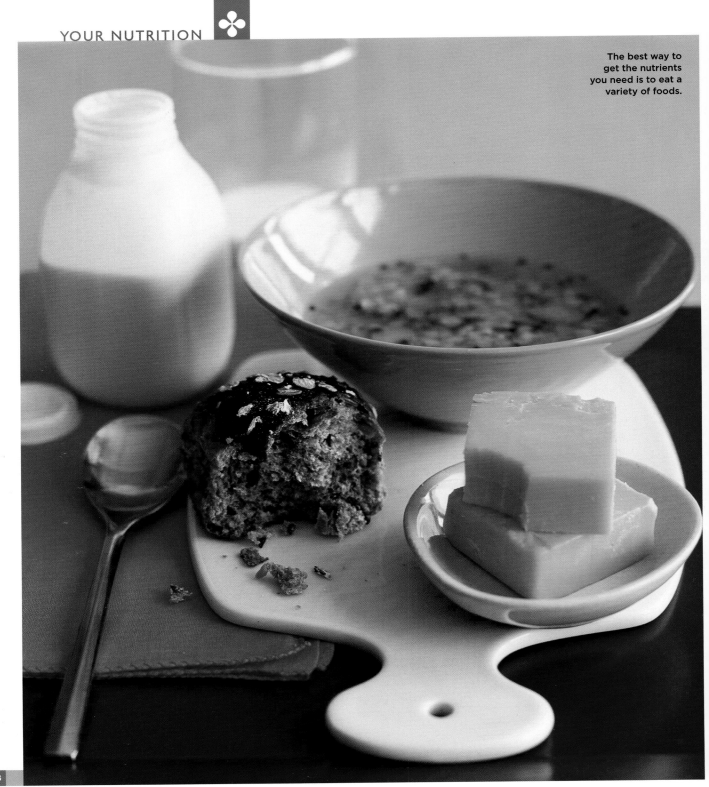

The best way to get the nutrients you need is to eat a variety of foods.

dinner

entree (pick 1)

Chicken-Apricot Curry With Rice*
Halibut With Grilled Corn and
   Tomato Salsa*
Black Bean and Couscous Salad*
Steak and potato: 3 ounces extra-lean
   grilled steak and a baked potato topped
   with 2 tablespoons sour cream.
Fettuccine with shrimp and vegetables:
   Sauté 2 garlic cloves, minced; 2 green
   onions, chopped; and 5 jumbo shrimp
   in 1 teaspoon olive oil, then mix and
   heat with 2 tablespoons dry white wine;
   3 tablespoons chicken broth; $1/2$ cup
   cooked broccoli; and $1/4$ cup cooked
   carrot rounds. Serve with 1 cup
   cooked fettuccine.
Tofu fajita: 1 10-inch flour tortilla filled with
   the following, grilled: 3 ounces tofu cubes,
   $1/4$ cup red onion slices, $1/4$ cup green
   pepper and $1/2$ cup shredded cabbage,
   tossed with 1 tablespoon fajita sauce.

calcium (pick 1)

1 cup vanilla soy milk, fortified with calcium
   and vitamin D
1 cup low-fat (2%) milk
6 ounces low-fat yogurt
1 ounce sharp cheddar cheese
$2/3$ cup low-fat milk blended with $1/4$
   teaspoon cinnamon, 1 tablespoon cocoa
   powder and 4 ice cubes

vegetables (pick 2)

1 cup steamed spinach, sautéed with
   1 minced garlic clove, 1 teaspoon olive oil
   and salt and pepper to taste
Sweet-potato "fries": 1 sweet potato, sliced
   into $3/4$-inch strips. Rub with 1 teaspoon
   olive oil and bake on a cookie sheet at
   400° F for 30 minutes or until cooked
   through.
Sautéed asparagus: 2 cups fresh asparagus
   spears sautéed in 2 teaspoons soy sauce,
   2 tablespoons chicken broth and garlic
   powder. Sauté 12–15 minutes, then top
   with thin lemon slices.
Tossed salad: $1 1/2$ cups lettuce; $1/2$ medium
   tomato, chopped; 1 tablespoon cooked
   kidney beans; and 1 tablespoon creamy
   cucumber salad dressing.
Corn and peppers: $1/2$ cup corn and $1/3$ cup
   diced sweet red peppers sautéed in
   1 teaspoon butter.
Gingered carrots: 1 cup steamed, sliced
   carrots tossed with $1/4$ teaspoon grated
   fresh ginger, 2 teaspoons orange
   marmalade and 1 teaspoon melted butter.

in 2nd & 3rd trimesters (pick 1)

2 slices French bread
1 cup steamed brown rice
1 cup frozen vanilla yogurt topped with
   $1/2$ teaspoon orange zest
1 cup decaffeinated cappuccino with
   1 biscotti

* Recipes are on the following page.

Your vitamin and mineral needs skyrocket during pregnancy, so you need to choose healthful, nutrient-rich foods whenever possible.

the recipes

Chicken-Apricot Curry With Rice (serves 4)

$^2/_3$ cup long-grain brown rice
1 tablespoon butter
$^2/_3$ cup chopped onion
3 garlic cloves, minced
$^1/_4$ cup diced celery or leeks
1 tablespoon curry powder
8 ounces skinless, boneless chicken breasts, cut into bite-size pieces
$^1/_3$ cup apricot preserves
1 medium apple, cored and cut into small pieces
$^1/_3$ cup water
$^1/_4$ cup golden raisins
Salt to taste
$1^1/_2$ cups plain low-fat yogurt
2 tablespoons cornstarch
$^1/_4$ teaspoon hot pepper flakes

Cook rice according to package directions without butter or margarine. Cover and keep warm.

In a large nonstick skillet, melt butter over medium heat. Add onion, garlic, celery, and curry powder and cook for 1 minute. Push mixture to the side of the skillet and add chicken; cook and stir for 5 minutes or until chicken is no longer pink. Stir in onion mixture from the sides. Stir in preserves, apple, water, raisins and salt.

In a small bowl, blend yogurt, cornstarch and pepper flakes; then stir into chicken mixture. Cook until mixture is thickened and bubbly, stirring constantly over medium heat. Simmer for 2 minutes, remove from heat and serve over rice.

Nutritional information per $1^1/_2$-cup serving: 350 calories; 15 percent fat (6 grams); 61 percent carbohydrates; 24 percent protein; 3.23 grams fiber; 196 milligrams calcium; 1.25 milligrams iron; 21 micrograms folic acid.

Halibut With Grilled Corn (serves 5)

1 lemon, sliced thin
1 cup white wine
5 garlic cloves, minced
$1^1/_2$ pounds fresh halibut, washed
2 large ears of corn, husked
Olive oil
4 large, firm tomatoes, diced
$^1/_3$ cup red onion, chopped
3 cloves garlic, minced
2 canned green chilies, drained and chopped
1 tablespoon fresh oregano, chopped
2 tablespoons fresh lime juice
3 tablespoons fresh cilantro, chopped
1 teaspoon olive oil
Salt to taste
$2^1/_2$ cups cooked brown rice

Mix lemon, wine and garlic; add halibut. Marinate 1-3 hours.

For salsa: Heat grill. Brush corn with olive oil; grill over medium heat until tender and blackened (about 7 minutes), turning often. Cut kernels from cob and place in a serving bowl. Add tomatoes, onion, garlic, chilies, oregano, lime juice, cilantro and 1 teaspoon olive oil. Mix and season with salt. Let stand for 15-30 minutes before serving.

Grill fish until done, but not dry (about 4 minutes on each side, depending on the thickness). Fish is done when firm and opaque. Place on a serving platter and top with salsa. Garnish with lemon slices. Serve immediately with brown rice.

Nutritional information per serving: 332 calories; 15 percent fat (5.5 grams); 45 percent carbohydrates; 40 percent protein; 5.1 grams fiber; 87 milligrams calcium; 2.38 milligrams iron; 55.5 micrograms folic acid.

Black Bean and Couscous Salad (serves 5)

3 teaspoons olive oil
5 tablespoons red wine vinegar
2 teaspoons Worcestershire sauce
3 garlic cloves, minced
$1^1/_2$ teaspoons ground cumin
3 cups canned black beans, drained
1 teaspoon fresh oregano, chopped
$2^1/_2$ tablespoons fresh lemon juice
$^3/_4$ cup chicken broth
3 cups cooked couscous
$1^1/_2$ cups green, red and orange peppers, chopped
$^2/_3$ cup fresh parsley, chopped
$^1/_2$ cup green onions, chopped
Salt and pepper to taste

Mix 2 teaspoons oil, $2^1/_2$ tablespoons vinegar, Worcestershire, 1 garlic clove and 1 teaspoon cumin in a large bowl. Add beans and mix. Refrigerate.

For dressing: In a large bowl, combine remaining vinegar, garlic and cumin, along with the oregano and lemon juice. Set aside.

For couscous: In a 1-quart pan, heat chicken broth and remaining olive oil until simmering. Stir in the couscous, cover and remove from heat. Let stand 5 minutes, then stir with a fork. Mix couscous into dressing and cool to room temperature.

Combine the bean mixture and couscous. Add peppers, parsley and green onions. Stir gently, adding salt and pepper, until ingredients are mixed well. Serve at room temperature.

Nutritional information per $^1/_4$-cup serving: 314 calories; 10 percent fat (3.62 grams); 70 percent carbohydrates; 20 percent protein; 11.7 grams fiber; 97 milligrams calcium; 4.57 milligrams iron; 137 micrograms folic acid.

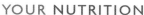

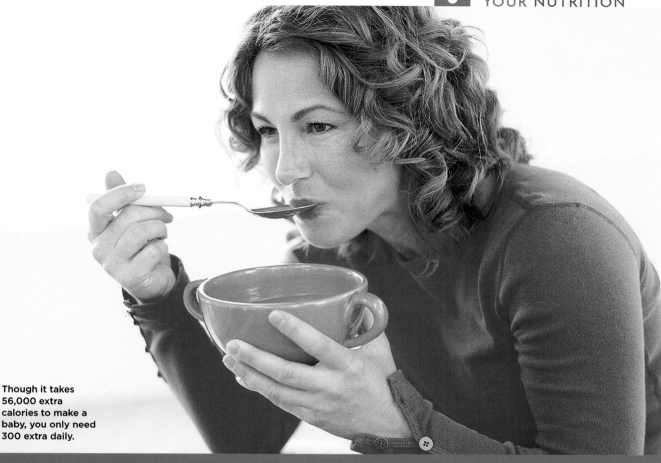

Though it takes 56,000 extra calories to make a baby, you only need 300 extra daily.

how much weight should you gain?

Your goal is to gain just enough weight, but not too much. (Stored body fat is not the stuff babies are made of!) Women of normal weight should aim to gain 25 to 35 pounds during pregnancy, underweight women should gain 28 to 40 pounds, and overweight women should gain 15 to 25 pounds. If you're carrying twins, aim for a weight gain of 35 to 45 pounds, according to a committee from the Institute of Medicine in Washington, D.C. You should pay attention to your weight before becoming pregnant, too. It has been shown that women who are very overweight when they conceive increase their risk of having babies with birth defects, according to the Centers for Disease Control and Prevention in Atlanta.

do's & don'ts

>>>IF YOU'RE LIKE MANY PREGNANT women, you vowed to eat healthier the minute you found out you were expecting. You may even have started making a mental list of nutritional do's and don'ts: Eat more calcium-rich foods, get more protein, cut out the caffeine and junk foods. Developing healthy eating habits will set the stage for your baby to grow into a strong child and adult, as well as ultimately reduce his risk for certain diseases. In fact, scientific research increasingly shows that a prenatal diet rich in nutrient-dense foods is key in preventing heart disease, diabetes, obesity and many types of cancer. Following are some rules to eat by for a healthy pregnancy.

DO choose foods that do double duty.
Nutrient-dense foods, such as yogurt, peanut butter, chicken, beef, eggs and dairy products, are high in protein, calcium and iron, all the nutrients your baby needs to grow and develop. Milk provides calcium and plenty of protein. Lean pork and beef contain protein, along with B vitamins, iron and zinc. Orange juice offers folate plus vitamin C and vitamin C, helps you absorb iron from foods such as fiber-rich black beans and spinach. Whole grains are filled with fiber, B vitamins, magnesium and zinc.

DON'T fill up on empty calories.
Candy, cake, cookies and ice cream definitely don't count as double-duty, nutrient-rich foods. It's OK to have them during pregnancy—but in moderation, says Rose Ann Hudson, R.D., L.D., co-author of *Eating for Pregnancy: An Essential Guide to Nutrition With Recipes for the Whole Family* (Marlowe & Co., 2003). "One of the ways we enjoy life is to eat foods that aren't high in nutrition, like desserts," she says. "Limit these foods to once a day, in the portion listed on the label; you won't feel deprived and you also won't overeat."

DO remember that you're not *really* eating for two.
"I recommend that women 'eat to appetite,'" says Karen Nordahl, M.D., a Vancouver-based family physician. This means you should eat until you are not hungry rather than until you are full. "Make healthy food choices and reduce or eliminate processed food," Nordahl adds. "Excessive weight gain is associated with longer labor, pregnancy-induced hypertension and gestational diabetes." Indeed, many moms-to-be don't realize that they need only 300 extra calories a day—and only in the second and third trimesters.

DON'T forget to take your prenatal vitamin.
A daily prenatal vitamin and mineral supplement acts as a safeguard, providing nutrients—vitamins, folate, iron and more—beyond what you'll get from meals and snacks. "In a perfect world, you'd get all your nutrients from foods," says Suki Hertz, M.S., R.D., a nutritionist and chef in New York. "But since our lives are often a little less than perfect, you should take a supplemental prenatal vitamin that contains 100 to 200 percent of the recommended dietary intakes."

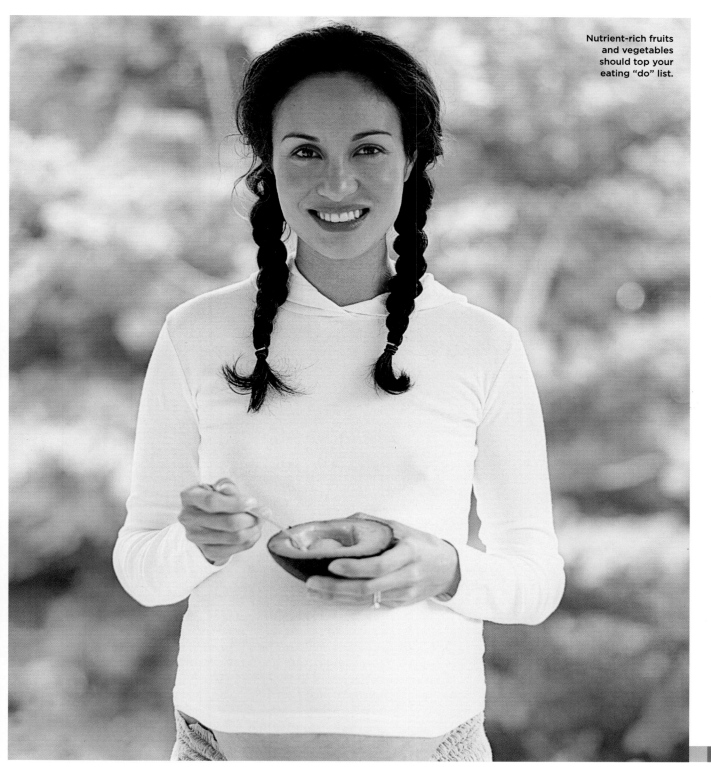

Nutrient-rich fruits and vegetables should top your eating "do" list.

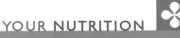

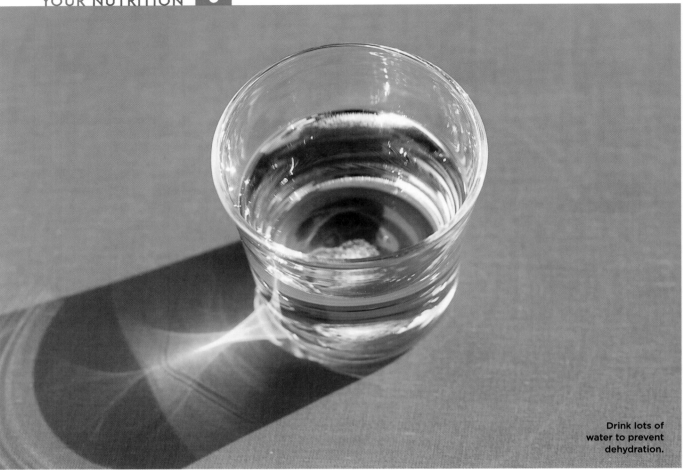

Drink lots of water to prevent dehydration.

DO focus on nutritional variety.

Along with taking your prenatal supplement, the best way to make sure that you'll get all the proper nutrients is to eat the following daily:

- 9 servings from the whole-grains group (bread, cereal, rice and pasta)
- 2–3 servings of protein-rich foods from the meat, poultry, fish, beans, eggs and nuts group
- 4 servings from the vegetable group
- 3 servings from the fruit group
- 3 servings from the milk, yogurt and cheese group.

DON'T neglect water and fiber-rich foods.

Drink plenty of liquids—at least eight glasses of water daily—to help prevent dehydration. "Without enough water, many of our regular body functions can't take place, including cell respiration, digestion and absorption of nutrients," Hudson says. But stay away from alcohol while pregnant; even small amounts have been linked to birth defects.

Fluids also will help prevent constipation, as will high-fiber foods such as whole-grain breads and pastas, and lots of fruits and vegetables. Aim for at least 25 to 35 grams of fiber every day (³/₄ cup of bran cereal, for example, contains an average of 5 grams of fiber).

DO avoid unpasteurized and certain uncooked foods.

These foods include unpasteurized soft cheeses such as brie, Camembert, feta, blue-veined and Mexican-style cheeses. They can harbor *Listeria,* a bacterium that can cause a serious infection and lead to premature delivery, infection in the newborn, miscarriage or stillbirth. Eating pasteurized cheeses is considered safe.

Deli meats also may pose a risk, so buy prepackaged cold cuts rather than those from the deli counter, or heat deli-counter meats to steaming hot before eating them. "To minimize the risk of listeriosis, cook all leftovers and deli foods to at least 140° F," Hertz says.

In addition, never eat raw or undercooked meat, sushi, seafood or eggs during pregnancy; they, too, can carry *Listeria.* And steer clear of fish that may contain excessive amounts of mercury, such as shark, king mackerel, tilefish and swordfish.

The March 2004 U.S. Food and Drug Administration guidelines recommend limiting low-mercury fish consumption to 12 ounces a week. Safe choices include canned light tuna, catfish, pollock, salmon and shrimp. (See "Fish Tales" on page 62.)

You can eat dessert-types of foods once a day. This way, you won't feel deprived or overeat.

how much is one serving?

Dairy	Protein	Fruits	Vegetables	Whole Grains
1 cup milk, soy milk or yogurt; 1½ ounces natural cheese; or 2 ounces processed cheese	2–3 ounces cooked lean meat, poultry or fish; ½ cup tofu; 2 eggs; or 2 tablespoons peanut butter	1 medium-size piece (such as an apple or banana), ½ cup chopped fruit, ½ cup cooked fruit (such as applesauce) or ¾ cup fruit juice	1 cup raw leafy vegetables, ½ cup raw or cooked vegetables, or ¾ cup vegetable juice	1 slice of bread, ½ cup cooked cereal (such as oatmeal) or ½ cup rice or pasta

the fab 5

>>>EACH YEAR, SCIENTISTS UNCOVER new information about the critical benefits of nutrients in a fetus's mental and physical development, including a reduced risk of birth defects and disease in newborns. Prenatal vitamins help, but they can't do the job alone, which is why diet is so important. Following are the five most important nutrients—and how much of each—you need daily to build a healthy baby.

1. CALCIUM 1,200 mg

Your developing baby needs this mineral for optimal bone growth. Getting enough calcium during pregnancy also can help prevent you from losing bone density and developing osteoporosis as you age. A day's worth of calcium: 1 cup fat-free milk, 1 cup instant fortified oatmeal, 1 ounce cheddar cheese, 1 cup low-fat yogurt and a salad with 1 cup chicory greens.

2. PROTEIN 60 g

The amino acids in protein are responsible for tissue growth and repair in your body as well as your baby's. "One way to get enough protein each day is to consume two 3-ounce servings of meat or fish, plus three servings of dairy products," says Lola O'Rourke, M.S., R.D., a spokeswoman for the American Dietetic Association. "For vegetarians, beans, eggs and nuts are good sources." Avoid fish with high mercury content such as shark, mackerel and swordfish; safer types such as wild salmon and flounder are OK—just don't limit your intake to one type. A day's worth of protein: 1 cup low-fat milk, 1 egg, 3 ounces turkey breast, $1/2$ cup baby lima beans and 3 ounces salmon.

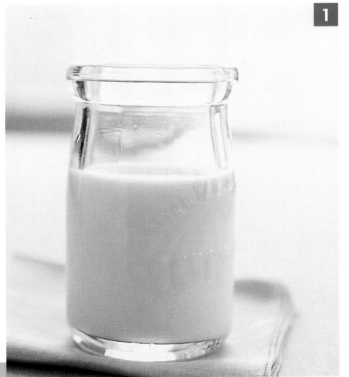

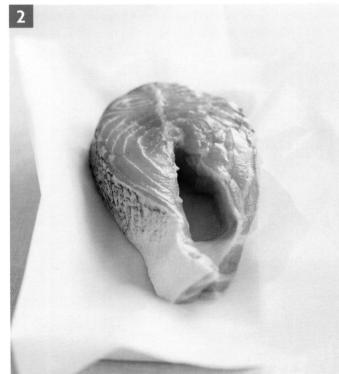

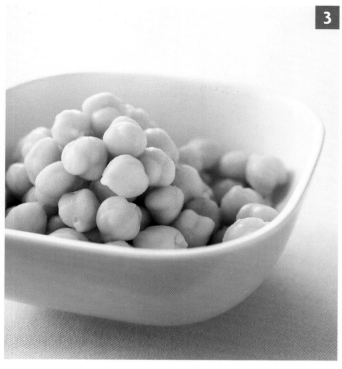

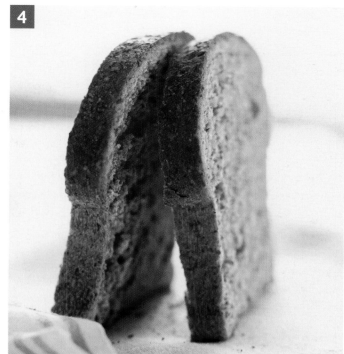

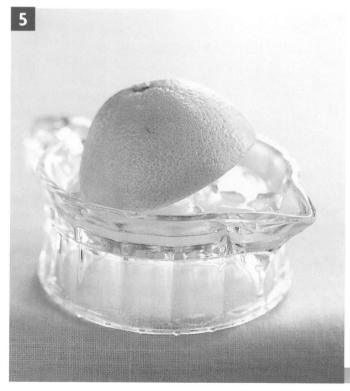

3. FOLATE 400 mcg

This B vitamin and its synthetic form, folic acid, protect against neural-tube defects, such as spina bifida. Because these defects develop in the first 28 days after conception, women need to eat foods rich in folate or fortified with folic acid and take a daily supplement *before* becoming pregnant. A day's worth of folate: 1 cup orange juice from concentrate, 1 cup fortified oatmeal and 1/2 cup chickpeas.

4. IRON 30 mg

Iron helps both your and your growing baby's blood transport oxygen throughout your bodies. It also plays an important role in proper muscle and organ function. A day's worth of iron: 1 cup fortified oatmeal, 2 slices whole-wheat bread, 3 ounces broiled beef tenderloin, 1 baked potato with skin and 2 cups cooked spinach.

5. VITAMIN C 70 mg

Vitamin C may help prevent preterm delivery. Researchers suspect this nutrient may be necessary for proper collagen formation, which is key to strengthening your body's membranes. You need a good amount of vitamin C to prevent premature rupture of the membranes, which causes preterm delivery. An analysis of 2,064 pregnant women showed that daily intakes of 21 mg or less during the first trimester doubled the risk of preterm delivery. A day's worth of vitamin C (choose one of the following): 1 cup strawberries, 1 medium navel orange or 1 cup broccoli.

what's safe to eat, what's not

>>> **NOW THAT YOU'RE EXPECTING,** every meal and snack provides the chance to supply you and your growing baby with the important nutrients you both need to be healthy. If you're like most pregnant women, you want to eat what's safest for your baby. Three top food-safety questions pregnant women ask concern organic foods, fish and mercury, and trendy dieting (e.g., low-carb/high-protein). Here, we hope to give you enough information so that you can decide for yourself—and for your baby, of course.

should you go organic?

The thought of pesticide residues, antibiotics and toxic chemicals lurking in your food probably didn't keep you up at night before you became pregnant. But now that you're eating for you and your baby, you may feel compelled to buy the safest foods available. In fact, a recent survey from The Hartman Group, a think tank in Bellevue, Wash., revealed that having children is the most significant trigger for "going organic." And, thanks to a burgeoning $9-billion-a-year industry, organic products are flooding the marketplace. The question is, now that such products are so readily available, is it time for you to go organic?

A QUESTION OF SAFETY

The hallmark of organic food is that it is grown via environmentally friendly farming techniques. In lieu of synthetic substances, natural fertilizers are used, as are biological predators like ladybugs to manage pests. To earn organic certification from the U.S. Department of Agriculture (USDA), farmland must be free from prohibited substances (pesticides, artificial fertilizers, etc.) for at least three years, and organic animal products must come from animals raised without hormones or antibiotics, explains Kathleen Merrigan, Ph.D., director of the agriculture, food and environment program at the Friedman School of Nutrition Science and Policy at Tufts University in Boston. But is organic food automatically better for you and your developing baby? That depends on who you ask.

A recent study from the University of California, Davis, found that organically grown berries and corn contain nearly 60 percent more polyphenolics, natural antioxidants that may improve your health. The theory: Crops grown without pesticides or herbicides produce more of these chemicals due to stress from insects or other pests, similar to the way humans build antibodies to ward off bacterial "bugs."

Even so, agencies such as the USDA and the American Dietetic Association stand behind their claims that organic foods are not nutritionally superior to or safer than conventionally produced foods. "There are no definitive studies that organic is better for you," Merrigan says. "Instead, we rely on intuition that food from an environmentally sound system is probably healthier." It's probably superior for your baby, too. Though no data suggest that food treated with antibiotics or pesticides will harm a fetus, several agencies have called for more studies on the long-term health effects of these substances.

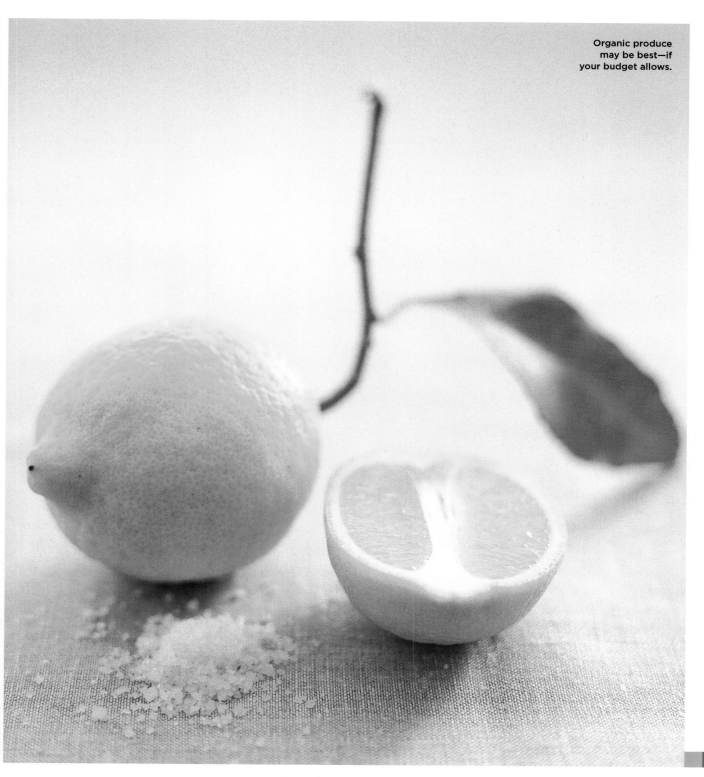

Organic produce may be best—if your budget allows.

Up to 80 percent of nonorganic processed foods like crackers and cookies contain a component, such as canola oil, from a genetically modified crop.

BEST BANG FOR YOUR ORGANIC BUCK

Despite the obvious environmental benefits and perceived health effects, expense may stand in the way of many women choosing to go "all organic." So the question becomes, which organic foods should you be buying?

As fruits and vegetables are the most pesticide-laden (see "The Dirty Dozen" at right), organic versions of these products now account for more than 40 percent of organic-food sales. Some produce such as apples and berries are more vulnerable to pests (and therefore more pesticide-protected) than "cleaner" produce like bananas, oranges and broccoli.

But despite the price (organic baby spinach usually costs about 50 cents more per pound; organic carrots, 20 cents more), an organic label doesn't guarantee that foods are pesticide-free. According to the USDA, 23 percent of organic produce contains pesticide residues. These chemicals can come from substances in the soil (some of which have been banned for decades but remain in the ground) or drift onto organic crops from nearby fields.

When it comes to livestock, conventionally raised animals are given hormones and antibiotics to prevent disease, enhance growth and increase milk production. Organically raised livestock don't receive such treatments, and their feed is all-organic.

While your baby is developing, you'll want to eat the best foods possible, and choosing organic food makes sense if your budget allows. But remember, the most important thing is to maintain a healthy diet during pregnancy without making yourself crazy in the process.

where to buy organic?

These days, you don't have to look far to find organic food (many supermarkets now stock organic). Here are three great shopping options:

1. Farmers markets The number of farmers markets featuring organic produce has nearly doubled since the government began tracking them in 1994; to find one near you, visit *www.ams.usda.gov/farmersmarkets/map.htm*.

2. Natural- or specialty-food stores Look for a Whole Foods (*www.wholefoods.com*), Wild Oats (*www.wildoats.com*) or Trader Joe's (*www.traderjoes.com*) store in your area.

3. Online grocers *www.diamondorganics.com* delivers to your door.

the dirty dozen

The top 12 most pesticide-laden foods when grown conventionally:

1. Peaches

2. Strawberries

3. Apples

4. Spinach

5. Nectarines

6. Celery

7. Pears

8. Cherries

9. Potatoes

10. Raspberries

11. Sweet bell peppers

12. Grapes (imported)

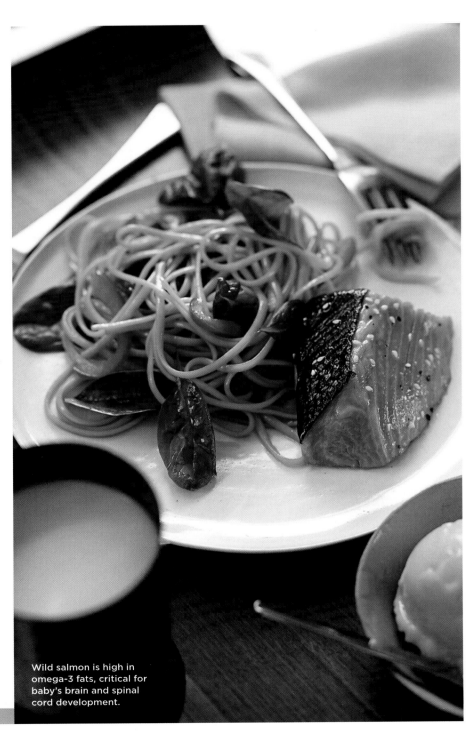

Wild salmon is high in omega-3 fats, critical for baby's brain and spinal cord development.

fish tales

Reports about the safety of fish, particularly regarding mercury, can leave pregnant women reeling. For years, however, doctors have touted the nutritional benefits of fish—it's an excellent source of good fats, lean protein and key nutrients. What's a pregnant woman to eat? Here, answers you've been waiting for.

Recent news stories about mercury poisoning may leave you wondering if fish is still such a healthy catch for you and your developing baby.

Mercury is a naturally occurring chemical from underwater volcanoes. It's also an industrial pollutant that has been linked to developmental delays and learning difficulties in children. And while nearly all fish contain some mercury, large predatory species such as shark, swordfish, king mackerel and tilefish contain the most. As a result, the standard advice is that pregnant or breastfeeding women and small children should avoid eating "big" fish.

A recent Harvard School of Public Health study found that children whose mothers eat large amounts of seafood high in mercury during pregnancy could suffer irreparable brain damage.

According to data from the Environmental Protection Agency (EPA), it is estimated that 630,000 babies in this country are born each year with high levels of mercury in their blood—more than double the previous estimate of 300,000 by the 1999–2000 National Health and Nutrition Examination Survey. The new estimate was based on recent research indicating that mercury in pregnant women tends to concentrate in umbilical-cord blood.

Fish that are lower in mercury: wild salmon, shrimp, canned light tuna, catfish and pollock.

A BALANCED PERSPECTIVE

Before you swear off fish altogether, some obstetricians and nutritionists argue that these findings do not necessarily reflect a danger for most moms-to-be in the United States. The Harvard study took place in Denmark's Faroe Islands, whose residents consume very large amounts of fish and whale meat, which are not common culinary fare in the States.

A report from the Office of Environmental Health Hazard Assessment found that people in the United States eat an average of 0.35 to 0.6 ounces of fish a day, approximately one meal a week. As for the EPA estimates, exceeding the safety level does not necessarily mean a baby's development will be impaired, since safe levels are set well below those known to show harm, says David Acheson, M.D., chief medical officer and director of Food Safety and Security at the U.S. Food and Drug Administration's (FDA's) Center for Applied Nutrition and Safety. Moreover, a recent study in the *Lancet* found no developmental defects in children born to women in the East African Seychelles islands, who ate an average of 12 fish meals a week while pregnant. And as for the increased mercury level in umbilical-cord blood, experts claim that it doesn't reflect the level in the fetus.

"We don't want to frighten people off of fish," says Edith Hogan, R.D., a Washington-based nutrition consultant. "Fish is a good source of high-quality protein and is low in saturated fat and loaded with nutrients like iron, zinc and calcium." And species such as salmon and tuna are high in omega-3 fatty acids, which are critical for develop-ment of the baby's brain and spinal cord. In addition, preliminary research suggests that a diet rich in omega-3 fatty acids may help decrease the chance of preterm birth.

THE RECOMMENDATIONS

The FDA and EPA agree that pregnant and breastfeeding women should limit their fish consumption to two or three meals per week (not to exceed 12 ounces total); avoid mercury-harboring species such as shark, swordfish, king mackerel and tilefish; and limit intake of bottom-feeders such as clams and other shellfish. "Pregnant women should eat medium-size, commercially sold fish like salmon and flounder," says Jonathan Scher, M.D., assistant clinical professor of obstetrics and gynecology at Mount Sinai Medical Center in New York. Check with your health department before eating fish caught in local rivers, lakes or streams to ensure that there are low levels of environmental toxins in the area.

What about canned tuna? Hogan says that the type used for canning comes from a smaller fish and doesn't have the same mercury profile as fresh tuna. In fact, FDA tests show that canned light tuna has a lower mercury level than canned albacore. To be safe, don't eat more than 6 ounces of albacore per week.

The bottom line: To protect you and your baby, eat different species rather than just one or a few types of fish. As with everything else, variety and moderation are key.

the lowdown on low-carb during pregnancy

If you've been cutting your intake of carbohydrates lately, you might be wondering if it's OK to do so throughout your pregnancy.

"Absolutely not," says Wahida Karmally, Dr.P.H., R.D., C.D.E., director of nutrition at the Irving Center for Clinical Research at Columbia University in New York. The only healthful diet recommended for pregnancy is a balanced one, she says.

To be more specific, when you cut carbs and increase protein intake, you put an extra burden on your kidneys, which already are working overtime during pregnancy. Limiting carb-containing foods also means cutting glucose, which your brain needs in order to function. You also may miss out on vital vitamins and nutrients (including fiber and antioxidants) that are essential for good health, Karmally explains. What's more, "you absolutely don't want to be in ketosis when you're pregnant," says Jodie Shield, M.Ed., R.D., a faculty member in the clinical nutrition department at Rush University in Chicago. Ketosis occurs in the absence of carbs, when the body burns its fat stores for fuel. As a result, the acid level in the blood spikes, much like it does when a person is starving or has untreated diabetes.

Going low-carb also can reduce the amount of folic acid (a B vitamin shown to reduce the risk of neural-tube defects) you get, since the main sources of folic acid in the typical American diet are fortified grain products such as cereals, breads and pastas—all big no-no's if you've sworn off carbs. This problem is compounded by the fact that foods naturally high in folic acid (including spinach and other fruits and vegetables) are allowed only in small amounts on some low-carb diets.

Rather than cutting the entire carb category, pregnant women should restrict their intake of processed foods made with refined sugars and flour and instead consume more nutritious carbs such as whole grains, fruits and vegetables. In short, Shield says, "when it comes to carbs, discriminate—don't eliminate."

When you cut carbs and increase protein intake, you put an extra burden on the kidneys, which are already working overtime in pregnant women.

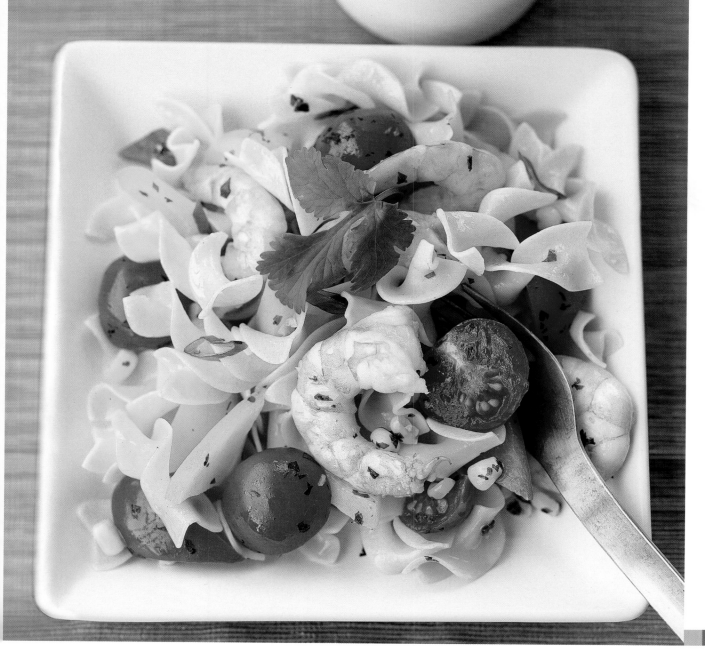

Don't cut
good carbs:
You'll miss
out on vital
nutrients.

the truth about baby weight

>>> **PREGNANT WOMEN OF NORMAL WEIGHT** should aim to gain 25 to 35 pounds, according to a committee from the Institute of Medicine. What you eat during these months will affect your pregnancy weight gain, as well as your post-pregnancy weight loss. Eat a healthy diet, and follow the nutrient guidelines in "Bottom Line" (opposite page) for the entire nine months.

Not all pregnant women gain weight the same way: Some women pack on the stubborn pounds all over, while others gain nearly all of it in their bellies and lose it practically the instant they give birth. The key is to think realistically, which, admittedly, can be difficult when we see a celebrity like Kate Hudson put on 60 pounds during her pregnancy (well over the recommended amount), then drop it all in a flash (OK, four months), thanks to twice-daily sessions with a personal trainer. But is such weight gain even healthy? And is such rapid weight loss a good idea?

Turns out, no and no. Gaining 60 pounds is too much, even if you're pregnant with twins, doctors say. Extreme weight gain can increase the chances of developing gestational diabetes and pregnancy-induced hypertension (especially if you're over 35), says Karen Nordahl, M.D., a Vancouver-based family physician and co-author of *Fit to Deliver* (Hartley & Marks, 2005), which covers exercise and pregnancy. Also to consider: A large weight gain could affect the size of the baby and complicate delivery.

Dropping pregnancy weight immediately after giving birth isn't a good idea if you're trying to nurse your baby, as you need extra calories and nutrients in order to keep producing breast milk. Even if you aren't nursing, it's not advisable to drop more than a pound and a half per week, says registered dietitian Karmally, who adds that if you lose weight any more rapidly, you'll also lose muscle mass.

Unless you have a personal trainer taking up residence at your house yelling at you to lift, lift, lift, that is. Needless to say, most of us don't. When you see the stunning "success" stories of celebrities, remember that it's their job to keep their bodies in top form—they have the time and the resources to hone their bodies to perfection.

Instead, take a more realistic approach. Watch what you eat, exercise on a regular basis and the weight will come off steadily, as it should.

bottom line

Choose from all the food groups every day so you get a variety of nutrients. Eat nine servings from the whole-grains group (bread, cereal, pasta); two to three servings of protein-rich foods (meat, poultry, fish, beans, eggs and nuts); seven servings from the fruit and vegetable group; and three servings from the dairy group.

Stay hydrated. Drink at least eight glasses of water daily (more during exercise) and avoid alcohol.

Eat nutrient-dense foods. To get the nutrients you need, including calcium, iron, folate and fiber, go for minimally processed foods such as yogurt, eggs, chicken and whole-grain cereals or breads.

Take a prenatal vitamin. Take a prenatal supplement that provides 100 percent to 200 percent of the daily recommended dietary intakes.

Avoid unpasteurized and uncooked foods. Certain foods may contain the *Listeria* bacterium that can cause infection and lead to premature delivery, infection in the newborn, miscarriage or stillbirth. Avoid unpasteurized soft cheeses and raw or undercooked meat, sushi, seafood or eggs.

Pay attention to your weight before pregnancy. Very overweight women are at increased risk of having babies with birth defects.

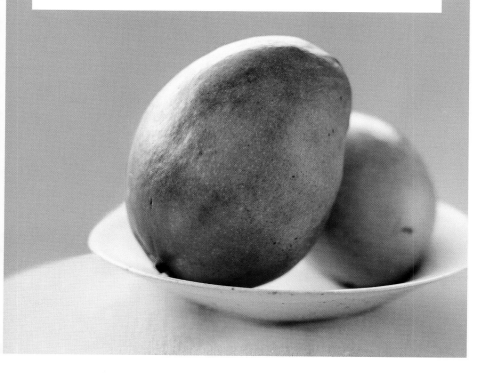

Q & A

>>>ANSWERS to your questions about prenatal nutrition and food safety.

Q I'm almost five months pregnant and I could eat creamed spinach for breakfast, lunch and dinner. Is a craving like this just a normal part of pregnancy or is it something I should worry about?

A Experiencing a food craving during pregnancy often indicates that a woman is deficient in an essential nutrient. The classic "pickles and ice cream" craving is likely the result of a need for additional calcium, and perhaps a secondary need to satisfy the salty and sour taste buds. The nutrient most women lack is iron and your craving for spinach, an iron-rich vegetable, certainly fits the bill. The cream in creamed spinach also may be soothing to a queasy stomach. As long as your craving is not an unhealthy one, pretty much any food is OK in moderation.

Q Before I became pregnant, I enjoyed an occasional glass of beer or wine or a martini. Now that I'm expecting, I was wondering if drinking alcohol can really hurt my baby?

A Yes. Drinking alcohol has been linked to fetal alcohol syndrome, a condition characterized by mental retardation, physical defects and behavioral problems, according to the March of Dimes. Instead, try fruit nectar mixed with seltzer or nonalcoholic sparkling cider. (Nonalcoholic beer contains trace amounts of alcohol and should be avoided.)

Q I can't start the day without my morning cup of java. What's the lowdown on caffeine?

A Although there is little evidence that moderate amounts of caffeine will harm your growing baby, research has shown that it can increase the baby's heartbeat, particularly in the last trimester. Also, consuming more than 300 milligrams of caffeine a day (the amount in two 5-ounce brewed cups) increases the risk of miscarriage, fetal growth problems and low birth weight. To be safe, switch to decaffeinated coffees, teas and colas, and drink smaller amounts, during your pregnancy.

Q I'm diabetic. Are sugar substitutes safe to eat now that I'm expecting?

A Based on years of research, sugar substitutes, such as saccharin and aspartame, appear to pose no health problems for pregnant women or their growing babies. If you do choose to include them in your diet, consider eating them in healthful foods, such as sugar-free yogurt, rather than in diet soft drinks, which contain no nutrients.

Q I've heard that I should stay away from soft cheeses. Which cheeses fit that description, and are they safe to eat if cooked, such as on a pizza or in a cheese sauce?

A Pregnant women should avoid soft cheeses because they also can contain *Listeria*. Brie, Camembert, Mexican-style cheeses (such as queso blanco), goat cheese and feta made with either cow's or sheep's milk all fall into the soft-cheese category. Even pasteurized soft cheeses are risky, says Erin Coffield, R.D., a registered dietitian with the New England Dairy and Food Council, because they tend to have a low pH level, which puts the cheese at risk for contamination. You should also avoid blue-veined cheeses such as Gorgonzola. If you do decide to eat soft cheese, be sure to heat it until it's bubbling hot.

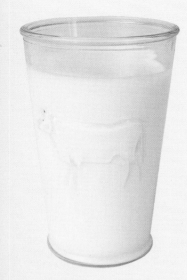

Q I hate milk, but I know I need calcium. What are some other sources to get the 1,000 milligrams I need daily?

A Try calcium-fortified orange juice or soy milk fortified with calcium and vitamin D, nutrition experts say. Other good sources of calcium include bok choy, white beans, canned salmon with bones, hard cheeses, yogurt and other low-fat dairy, and fortified oatmeal, such as Quaker Instant Oatmeal Nutrition for Women.

Q I'm a vegetarian. Can I get all the nutrients I need without eating beef, chicken and fish?

A Yes, as long as you make sure you get enough vital nutrients such as calcium, iron, zinc, vitamin D and the B vitamins, says Elizabeth Somer, M.A., R.D., author of *Nutrition for a Healthy Pregnancy* (Henry Holt and Co., 2002). Eggs, milk products, legumes, whole soy foods, vegetables and nuts are all excellent sources of these nutrients.

Q I love pâté and smoked salmon, but my friend told me I should avoid them now that I'm pregnant. Is she right?

A Pâté and foie gras made from undercooked goose or duck liver should not be eaten when you are pregnant because these foods could contain *Listeria,* says Keith-Thomas Ayoob, Ed.d, R.D. The FDA also warns pregnant women against eating refrigerated smoked seafood, such as salmon, trout, whitefish, cod, tuna and mackerel (often labeled as nova-style, lox, kippered, smoked or jerky), because they are cured, not cooked. However, canned versions of these foods are considered safe, as is vegetable pâté.

Q I'm excited about being pregnant, but I've got morning sickness all day, every day, and greasy foods make me feel worse. Is there anything I can eat to alleviate the nausea?

A "Morning sickness is a universal problem without a universal answer," says Miriam Erick, M.S., R.D., senior perinatal dietitian at Brigham and Women's Hospital in Boston and author of *Managing Morning Sickness* (Bull Publishing, 2004). "One food does not fit all." What alleviates one woman's nausea may not help you. That said, ginger and citrus fruits help many women, as do dry, salty foods, such as crackers and pretzels. Starchy foods like rice and potatoes may also help; you can boost their nutrient content by folding in vegetables.

Q I've read that pregnant women aren't supposed to eat soy food products. Is this true?

A Controversy has arisen recently because a small study showed that when pregnant female rats were fed a diet enhanced with genistein, a substance found in soybeans, the male offspring developed reproductive problems. Although further research is under way, many health experts (including Elizabeth Somer, M.A., R.D., and Johanna Dwyer, D.Sc., R.D., a professor at the Friedman School of Nutrition Science and Policy at Tufts University in Boston) feel you can enjoy soy foods such as tofu and soy milk in moderation (one serving per day) when you are expecting.

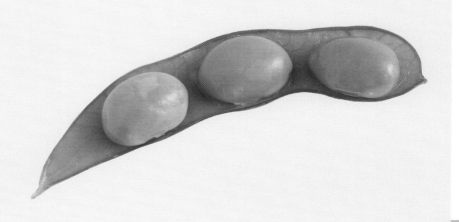

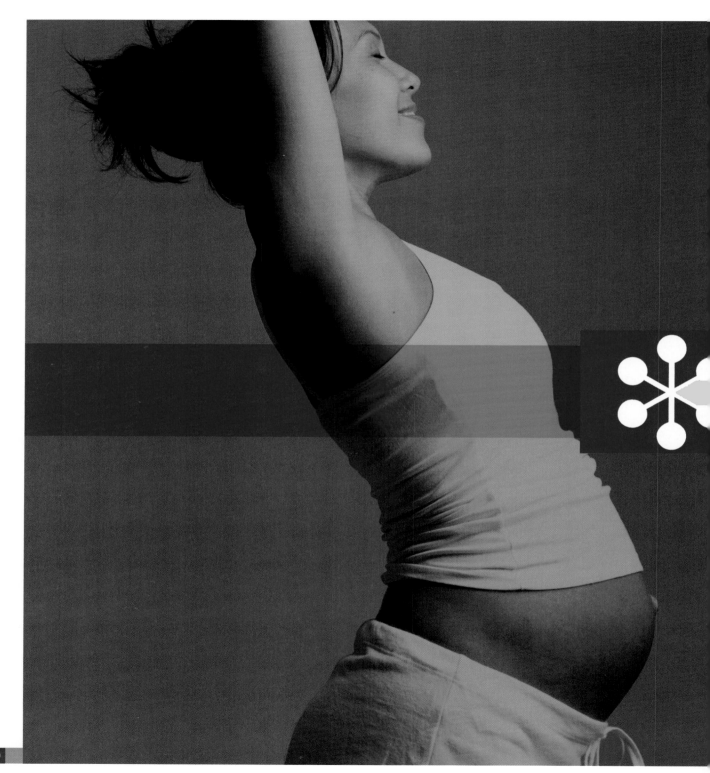

your health

Taking charge of your physical and mental health benefits both you and your baby. Here's how to avoid complications and have a happy 9 months.

>>> THERE HAS NEVER BEEN a better time to have a baby. The vast majority of infants in the United States are born healthy, most mothers experience no serious problems during pregnancy and many, if not most, deliveries are medically uneventful. Folic acid has been proven to help prevent several serious birth defects, and doctors have even learned to successfully treat certain disorders in babies while they're still in the womb.

Still, we could be doing better. For example, the percentage of babies born prematurely—at less than 37 weeks gestation—rose to 12 percent in 2002, the highest level in two decades. In the past 10 years, gestational diabetes rates have increased 35 percent. And today, 26 percent of babies are delivered by C-section, compared with only 5.5 percent in 1970. While a growing number of those procedures are elective, many of them are unplanned.

Overall, however, we know more than ever about how to have healthy babies, happy pregnancies and (relatively) easy deliveries. On the following pages we detail how to make this happen for you.

your body

>>> PREGNANCY CHANGES EVERYTHING, as you're well aware by now. On these pages about "Your Body," we provide a head-to-toe look at the pregnant body, starting with how you need to nurture it even before you conceive. So sit back, put your feet up and learn how to take good care of your baby's first home: your own body.

build a healthy baby

Boost the odds of giving birth to a healthy baby several months before you conceive. Here are tips from Siobhan M. Dolan, M.D., assistant medical director of the March of Dimes:

>**Take folic acid** Women who begin taking 400 micrograms of folic acid supplements daily starting one month before they conceive reduce their risk of having a baby with neural-tube defects, such as spina bifida, by 50 percent to 70 percent.

>**Treat infections before conceiving** Common health conditions like gum infections and bacterial vaginosis can increase the risk of prematurity and other problems. All infections should be treated and other health issues, such as diabetes, anemia and high blood pressure, should be brought under control before you get pregnant.

>**Start out at a healthy weight** Weighing either too much or too little can impair fertility and increase your risk of developing pregnancy complications. "The goal is to be neither too heavy nor too light," Dolan says. Aim for a body-mass index (BMI) of between 20 and 25 before becoming pregnant. (A 5-foot-4-inch woman who weighs 145 pounds has a BMI of 25.)

>**Schedule a preconception visit** Your OB-GYN or midwife will make sure you're healthy enough to get pregnant and review any prescription drugs you may be taking. If there's a chance you are at risk for having a baby with sickle-cell anemia, cystic fibrosis or other genetically linked diseases, get a referral to a genetic counselor to learn more about your risk and whether there are ways to reduce it.

>**Clean up your act** Avoid tobacco (secondhand smoke, too), alcohol and recreational drugs, all of which can contribute to prematurity, low birth weight and birth defects. Stop using over-the-counter remedies, including herbal supplements, unless they're approved by your doctor.

>**Seek support** It's easier to meet the demands of motherhood when you have a support system in place long before you deliver. Enlist the help of family and friends, meet other women who are considering pregnancy, start practicing stress-relief strategies such as meditation or yoga and get professional help, if needed, for emotional problems.

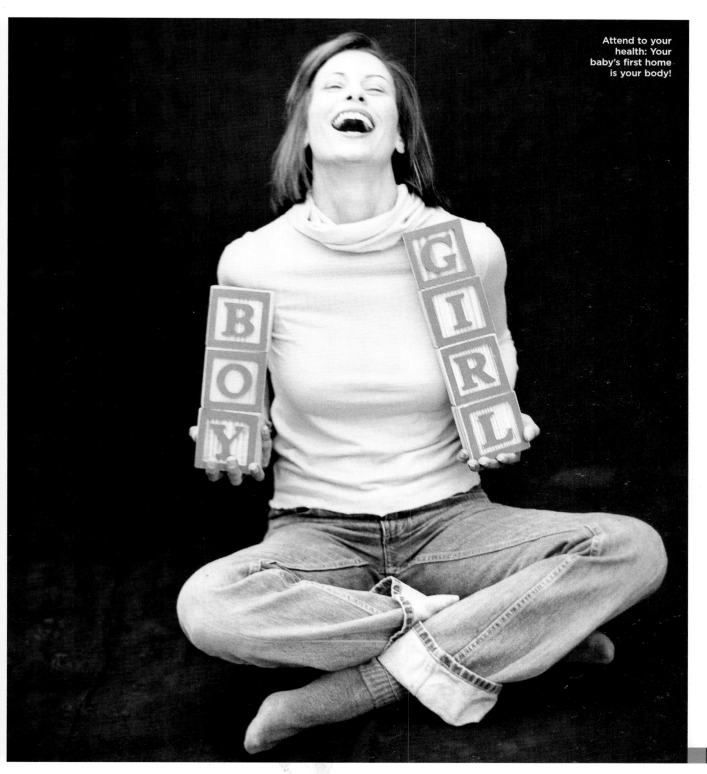

Attend to your health: Your baby's first home is your body!

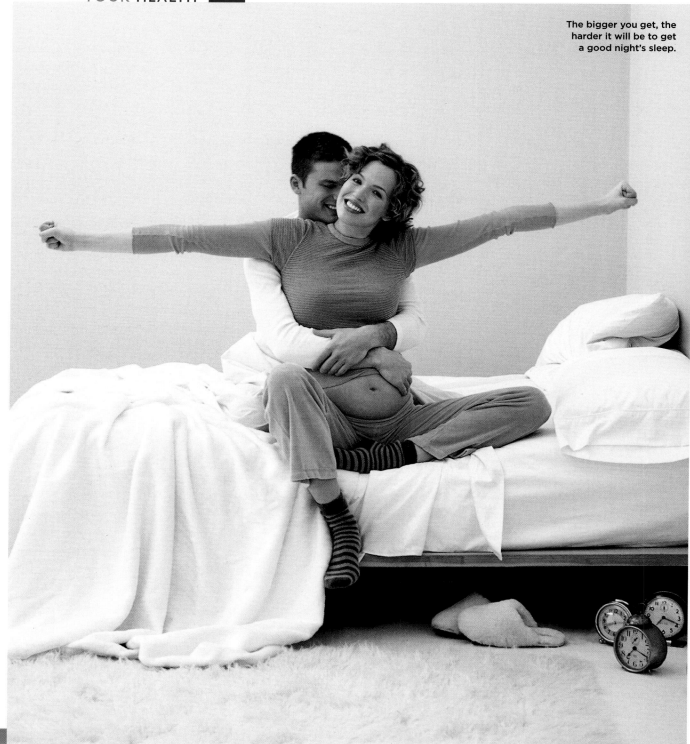

The bigger you get, the harder it will be to get a good night's sleep.

things that happen in bed

Sex >> During pregnancy it's generally safe, says Mary Herlihy, M.D., an assistant professor of obstetrics and gynecology at the University of Massachusetts Medical School in Worcester. The fetus is well protected from pokes and germs. However, your doctor may want you to abstain if you had a miscarriage in the first or second trimester of an earlier pregnancy, or if you have a history of premature delivery or ruptured membranes, are pregnant with twins or more, or have unexplained bleeding or placenta previa (a condition in which the placenta covers all or part of the cervical opening).

You can keep having sex until you go into labor unless your doctor has told you not to; however, your interest in it may vary widely over the course of your pregnancy. In the first trimester, nausea, hormonal changes, fatigue and breast tenderness can contribute to a decreased libido. Fortunately, it often rebounds with vigor in the second trimester, a time often referred to as the "honeymoon period" of pregnancy. Lovemaking may become more difficult later on as your growing belly gets in the way. Try different positions—on top, on your hands and knees, on your side—or have oral sex. When desire wanes, opt for sensual mutual massages or cuddling instead.

Sleep >> One of the first physical changes you may notice after you become pregnant is exhaustion. That extreme fatigue generally subsides somewhat in the second trimester, when, for most women, sleep comes easily and energy increases.

A good night's rest often proves elusive during the third trimester, however. "You may have a lot of aches and pains that you didn't have before," says Joan McCarthy, M.D., assistant professor of obstetrics and gynecology at the University of South Florida College of Medicine in Tampa. And as your belly grows, you'll find it difficult to lie on your stomach. At the same time, it's best not to sleep on your back because your uterus can press on the vein that returns blood from your lower body to your heart (the inferior vena cava). Heartburn may wake you up and, thanks to pressure on your bladder from your growing uterus, you'll likely need to urinate several times a night.

To get more comfortable, lie on your left side with a pillow under your belly and another one between your knees. Or try using either a large body pillow or a "maternity pillow" that supports your back and belly at the same time. (Both types are sold online at sites such as *www.bigvpillow.com;* or try the new Cuddle Pillow by Boppy, *www.boppy.com.*)

Both partners' desire levels can change dramatically over the course of the pregnancy.

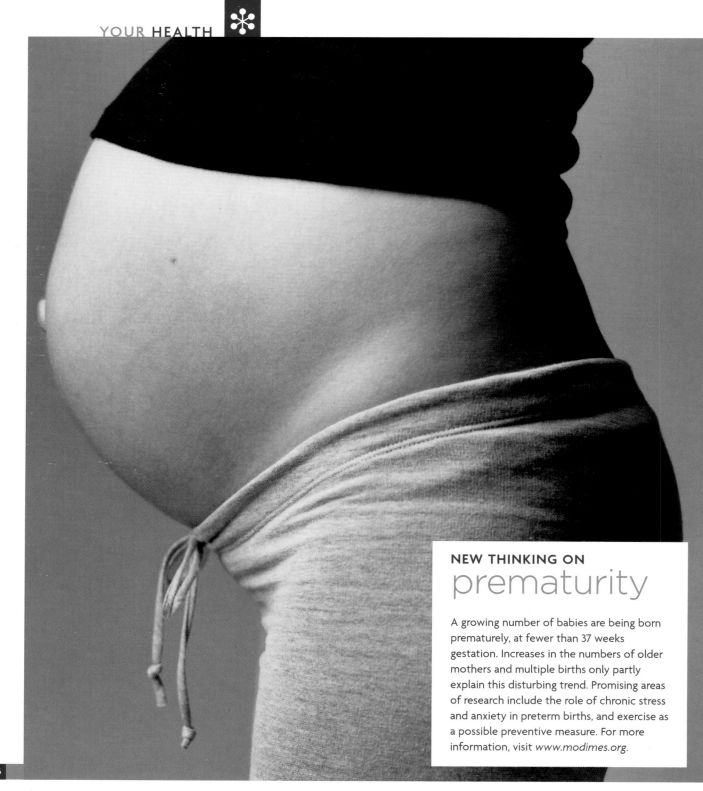

NEW THINKING ON
prematurity

A growing number of babies are being born prematurely, at fewer than 37 weeks gestation. Increases in the numbers of older mothers and multiple births only partly explain this disturbing trend. Promising areas of research include the role of chronic stress and anxiety in preterm births, and exercise as a possible preventive measure. For more information, visit *www.modimes.org*.

what can go wrong

Call your doctor if the baby's movements decrease markedly or if you have any signs of preterm labor, most notably, contractions. Also call if you experience bleeding or leaking of fluid from your vagina, severe headache, excessive swelling in your face or hands, sudden weight gain, blurred vision or constant and/or severe abdominal pain.

CONDITION/ INCIDENCE	WHAT IT IS	RISK FACTORS	PREVENTION	TREATMENT
MISCARRIAGE 15% of recognized pregnancies	Loss of fetus before 20 weeks (usually in first 12 weeks). Most result from chromosomal abnormalities in the embryo.	Possibly infections; hormonal and metabolic disorders; environmental exposures such as tobacco, drugs, alcohol.	Many not preventable; avoiding smoking and medications not cleared by your doctor may reduce the risk.	None needed if before about 8 weeks; later, D&C (dilatation and curettage) may be necessary.
PRETERM LABOR 12% of pregnancies	Labor that occurs before 37th week.	Multiple pregnancy; previous preterm birth; certain uterine or cervical abnormalities.	Do not use tobacco, alcohol or illegal drugs; have infections treated; get regular prenatal checkups.	Medications and rest sometimes stop labor long enough to give drugs that can help prepare baby for birth.
PREECLAMPSIA (also called toxemia) 5% of pregnancies	Blood pressure rises; protein collects in urine.	Chronic high blood pressure, kidney disease or diabetes; multiple pregnancy; overweight	None known, though exercise may help.	Bed rest, medication or induction of labor, depending on severity.
GESTATIONAL DIABETES 3%–5% of pregnancies	Body does not produce enough insulin, resulting in excess blood sugar.	Obesity; family history of diabetes; previous baby weighed more than 9 pounds.	Begin pregnancy at ideal weight; exercise; avoid excess weight gain during pregnancy.	Exercise and diet changes; sometimes insulin; condition generally disappears after delivery.
PLACENTA PREVIA 0.5% of pregnancies	Placenta covers all or part of internal opening of cervix.	More common in women who smoke, use cocaine or are over age 35.	Do not use tobacco, alcohol, drugs or herbal supplements not approved by your doctor.	Often corrects itself; C-section may be necessary to avoid severe bleeding.

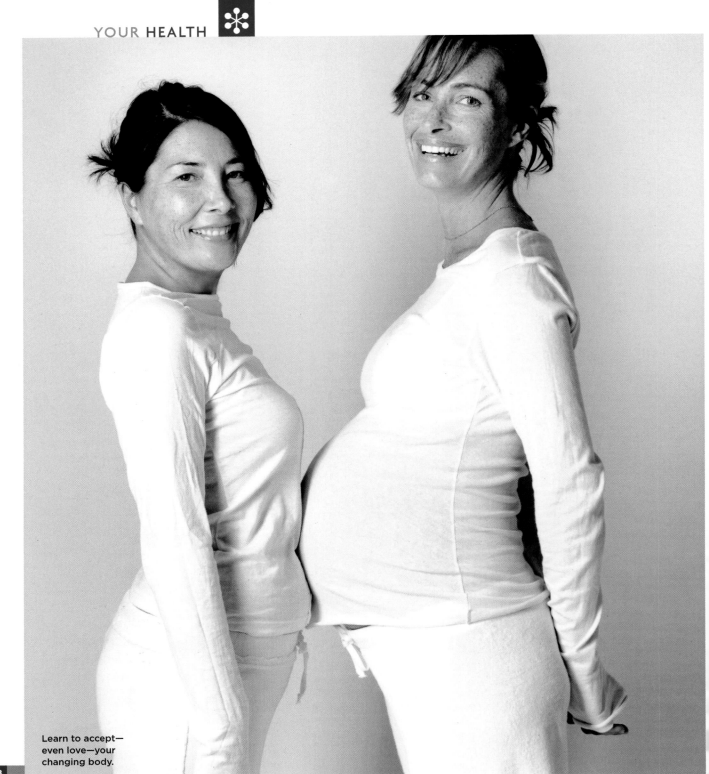

Learn to accept—
even love—your
changing body.

how your body will change

Here's a guide to some of the most common physical changes of pregnancy. Not only are they normal, but most will go away after your baby is born.

face and head

CHANGES Brownish, blotchy patches (melasma, or "the mask of pregnancy") develop around your eyes, nose and cheeks. Your face may look puffy, particularly in the last trimester (tell your doctor if you have severe swelling). You may become lightheaded as blood volume and vessel size increase and blood pressure decreases.

RELIEF Avoid exposure to sunlight. Lie on your left side (so the fetus doesn't press on a major blood vessel); drink plenty of water and avoid salty foods. Stand up slowly after you've been sitting or lying down.

breasts

CHANGES Breast tenderness often is the earliest noticeable change and can continue throughout pregnancy. Breasts may grow two or three cup sizes. Your nipples and areolas may get darker, veins and stretch marks may appear and skin may feel tight and itchy.

RELIEF Wear a soft, supportive bra. Apply moisturizer to damp skin after showering.

belly

CHANGES Nausea and vomiting are common in the first trimester. Acid reflux (heartburn) may start midpregnancy. A dark line (linea nigra) often develops from navel to pubic bone. Skin becomes tight.

RELIEF Nibble on crackers or toast before rising from bed; eat smaller, more frequent meals; try acupressure bands and ginger. Take antacids (with doctor's approval); don't eat just before bedtime.

back

CHANGES As your uterus grows and your center of gravity shifts, added strain is placed on your lower back, causing pain.

RELIEF Get massages from a prenatal-massage therapist; take daily walks; apply heat or ice; wear low-heeled (not flat), supportive shoes; sleep on your left side; try wearing an abdominal-support garment.

legs & feet

CHANGES Swelling and pain may occur, particularly as your uterus expands. Varicose veins can develop in the second or third trimester. Painful leg cramps may wake you up at night.

RELIEF Limit salty foods; rest with your legs elevated. Avoid sitting or standing for long periods; try support stockings. Stretch legs before going to bed; avoid pointing your toes.

butt & lower belly

CHANGES Constipation can start in the first trimester. Hemorrhoids (swollen veins in the rectum) may develop, particularly if you're constipated. The need to urinate increases in the first trimester, subsides in the second, then increases again during the third.

RELIEF Exercise; drink lots of water; eat foods high in fiber. Take warm baths and use doctor-approved, over-the-counter hemorrhoid creams or pads. Avoid drinking large amounts just before bedtime.

your mind

>>> NOW THAT YOU'VE HAD A TOUR of the pregnant woman's body, it's time to get inside her head as well. Here, we provide insight into your evolving emotions, relationships and identity. If you're wondering why you're thinking and feeling the way you are, you'll find all the mysteries revealed here.

out with your old life, in with the new

When you're pregnant, you're apt to feel happy, sad, hopeful, sentimental, depressed, joyful, guilty, excited, resentful, ecstatic, doubtful, confused, confident, anxious, blissful and fearful—all within the space of about five minutes.

It's perfectly normal for a pregnant woman to be on cloud nine one minute and in tears the next. "You move from one feeling to the other very rapidly as your life changes irrevocably," says Diana Dell, M.D., director of the maternal wellness program at Duke University Medical Center in Durham, N.C., and assistant professor in the departments of psychiatry and OB-GYN.

Indeed, a lot happens between that positive pregnancy test and the birth of a child. "Numerous profound and life-changing transformations go on during pregnancy," says Ellen Sue Stern, author of *Expecting Change: There's More to Pregnancy Than Having a Baby* (Meadowbrook Press, 2004). The relationship between you and your husband or partner can deepen as your priorities shift and you make space in your lives for another person. You also begin the emotional separation from your free-and-easy childless life; your body grows and transforms; you face career decisions; and you wonder about what kinds of parents you and your partner will be.

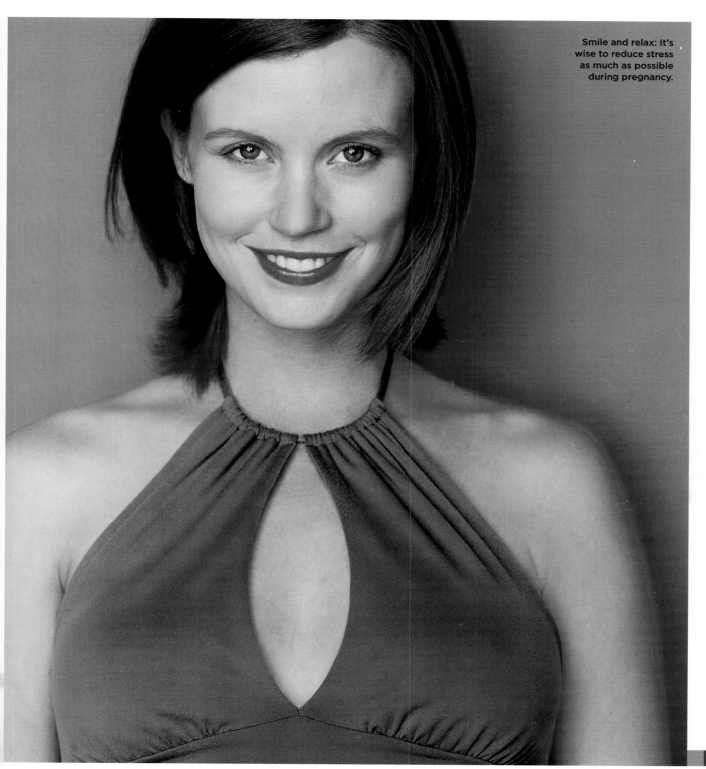

Smile and relax: It's wise to reduce stress as much as possible during pregnancy.

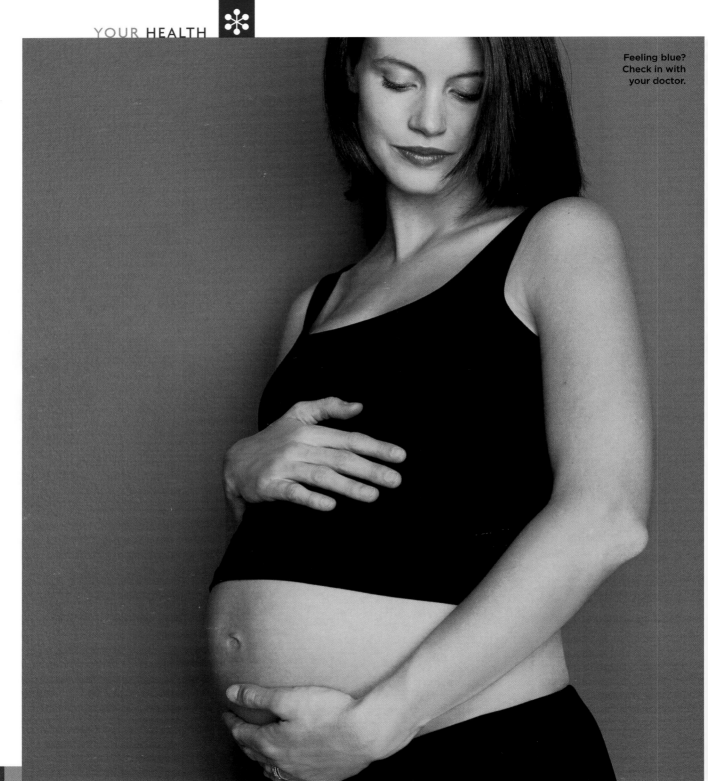

Feeling blue?
Check in with
your doctor.

when depression darkens a pregnancy

We think of pregnancy as a joyful time, but for some women it is just the opposite. "Pregnancy doesn't protect against depression," says psychiatrist and obstetrician Diana Dell, M.D., in Durham, N.C.

In fact, as many as 20 percent of pregnant women experience symptoms of depression. But few get help for it, according to a study conducted at the University of Michigan Depression Center in Ann Arbor. "Doctors used to think of pregnancy as a honeymoon away from the risk of depression, but this is turning out to be a myth," says study co-author Sheila Marcus, M.D., a clinical assistant professor of psychiatry at the university's medical school.

Prenatal depression is more likely to strike if a woman has a history of depression, if her pregnancy was unplanned or mistimed, if she is having marital problems or if she is suffering from medical complications. "We see a lot of women who are on bed rest become depressed," Dell says.

It's crucial that pregnant women who are suffering from depression be treated: Research shows that women who are depressed during pregnancy have a higher risk of postpartum depression. Furthermore, their babies aren't as healthy as other infants. Depression can be treated with psychotherapy, medication or both.

Dell points out that certain antidepressant drugs appear safe to use during pregnancy. Some mood stabilizers are associated with birth defects, however, so be sure to tell your doctor that you're pregnant before she prescribes any medication.

dealing with your changing body

Body-image issues tend to surface during pregnancy, as women in our society grow up surrounded by images that endorse thinness. Even if a woman recognizes that it's healthy and necessary during pregnancy, gaining weight can cause distress. "Women feel out of control when their body changes," says Catherine Chambliss, Ph.D., chairwoman of the psychology department at Ursinus College in the Philadelphia area. "It's hard to set aside all of that earlier programming."

On the other hand, some expectant moms learn to accept and even love their bodies like never before. In fact, "some women feel a real heightened sexuality during pregnancy," says Ellen Sue Stern, author of *Expecting Change: There's More to Pregnancy Than Having a Baby* (Meadowbrook Press, 2004).

If you're worried or apprehensive about anything related to pregnancy or impending parenthood, be sure to talk with someone—your spouse, your mom or a good friend. If you think you may need some extra help, discuss your concerns with your doctor or midwife or with a therapist.

the many moods of pregnancy

Hormonal changes are believed to contribute to the emotional ups and downs that occur during pregnancy, says Charles J. Lockwood, M.D., chairman of the department of obstetrics, gynecology and reproductive sciences at Yale University School of Medicine in New Haven, Conn. For example, levels of corticotropin-releasing hormone (CRH), which is known to induce anxiety, increase during pregnancy, peaking at the time of delivery. Progesterone levels also rise, and this hormone affects different women in different ways. For some, it behaves as a sedative (which would explain why some pregnant women feel so sleepy). In others, it promotes anxiety and depression.

Of course, the emotions of pregnancy aren't all negative. Some women report increased feelings of calm, optimism and enthusiasm. Here are the primary emotions you're likely to feel while you're expecting:

JOY/EXCITEMENT

If you and your spouse planned the pregnancy, your happiness probably began the very moment your pregnancy test read positive. For 80 percent of women, pregnancy is, overall, a time of joy, positive anticipation and excitement.

SADNESS/REGRET

It's not unusual to experience a kind of mourning period as you think about the life you are leaving behind. Pregnancy also may stir up feelings of sadness about a parent, sibling or friend who has died and thus can't share your pregnancy or meet your baby.

STRESS

This can be a particularly stressful time for many reasons: Your pregnancy was unplanned; you're facing financial, work or marital problems; you don't feel well; you're suffering pregnancy complications; you have a history of miscarriage or premature birth.

ANXIETY/WORRY

It's normal to feel anxious about your impending new responsibilities. You also may feel anxious about your job as you decide whether you'll return to work after your baby is born. Likewise, if you decide to stay home, you may worry about losing an income and interrupting your career.

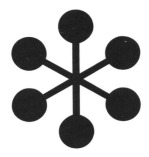

For 80 percent of women, pregnancy is, overall, a time of joy and excitement.

A FAMILY IS BORN

Every expecting couple worries about whether labor will go smoothly, if their baby will be healthy and if they will be good parents. This anxiety can express itself as bickering or avoidance, especially if it's kept bottled up inside.

A couple also may wonder how their relationship will change when they become parents. Even when they both look forward to having a baby, there can be an unspoken concern about sharing their affection. The woman may wonder if her partner will help out and provide emotional support for her and if he's really willing to do what's necessary to be a good father. And the man is most likely to worry about whether his partner will be so focused on the baby that she'll pay much less attention to him. The solution can be to talk about these fears.

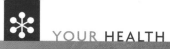

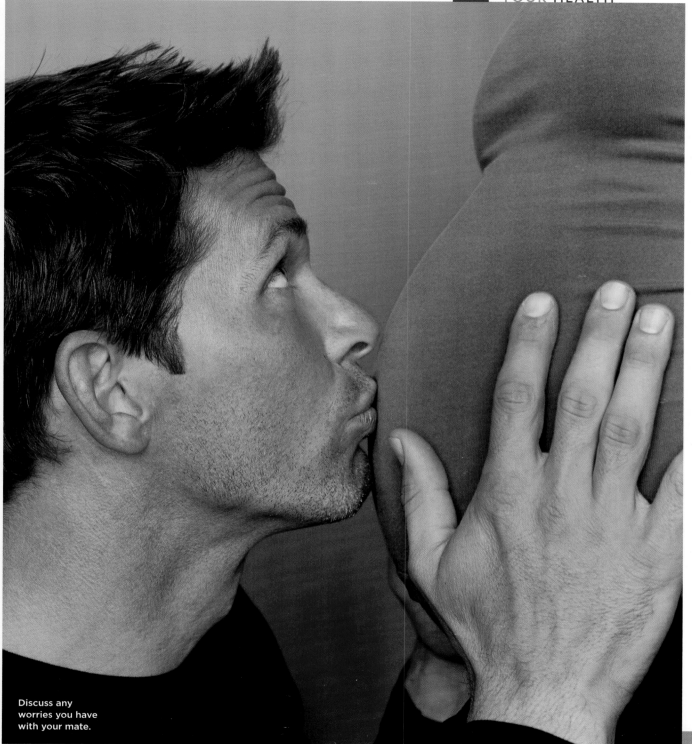

Discuss any
worries you have
with your mate.

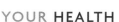
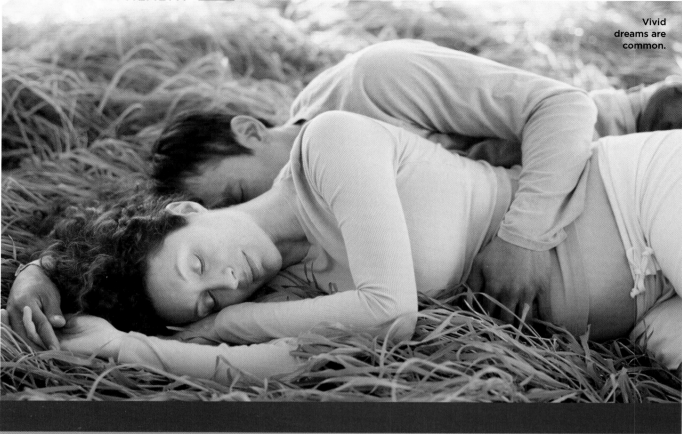

Vivid dreams are common.

pregnancy dreams what they mean

Vivid dreams are common during pregnancy. Here's a trimester-by-trimester guide, as explained by Raina Paris, Ph.D., a Beverly Hills, Calif., therapist and the author of *Mother-to-Be's Dream Book: Understanding the Dreams of Pregnancy* (Warner, 2000).

First trimester: Women tend to dream of the past—of their childhoods, lost loves, old boyfriends. "These are dreams of the life the woman had before she was pregnant," Paris says. They are a way to let go of her old identity.

Second trimester: Moms-to-be may dream of animals because they are bonding with their babies in an instinctive, almost animal-like way. They also may have dreams about the baby's gender, looks or personality. Anxiety-related dreams may occur, too.

Third trimester: Women may dream of swimming deep underwater or delving into caves. This signifies going deep inside oneself to prepare for giving birth, Paris says. Dreams of starring in a show or cooking an elaborate dinner reflect feeling like a creator.

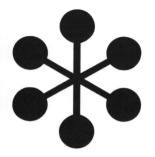

An expectant father may dream about being a hero or even winning the lottery because he is subconsciously celebrating his manhood.

how pregnancy affects your relationships

SEX COULD GET SEXIER Both partners' desire levels can change dramatically during the course of the pregnancy. Some women withdraw sexually, either because of their growing size or because their libido declines. Others feel aroused in an entirely new way, perhaps because they are enjoying the freedom of intercourse without birth control or because pregnancy is teaching them to enjoy their bodies in a new way. A man may find his wife sexier than ever, or he may be afraid to make love to her for fear he'll hurt the child. He also may fail to share his wife's excitement about the baby.

YOUR PARENTS WILL BECOME GRANDPARENTS Expecting a baby can alter a pregnant woman's relationship with her own parents. If you have had problems with your parents, pregnancy can facilitate healing, though experts warn that you shouldn't necessarily expect an instant reconciliation. Your pregnancy also can invite conflict, particularly if your mother (or father) is overly involved and offers endless unsolicited advice.

THINGS MAY CHANGE AT WORK Most of your co-workers probably will be supportive, but some may feel that you're not doing your fair share because you are tired, aren't feeling well or are missing work because of doctors' appointments. They also may be concerned that more tasks will fall on them during your maternity leave. If you sense that your co-workers are feeling shortchanged, try to make amends by thanking them for doing extra work and offering to help them out when you do feel rested and energetic.

YOUR FRIENDSHIPS WILL EVOLVE Relationships with your friends—particularly childless ones—may be put to the test during pregnancy. You may not have much in common anymore, particularly if your friends want to go out and party and you'd rather curl up at home and read parenting books. If this happens, it's important to sit down and explain to your friends that they're still important to you, but that, at least for a while, your priorities are changing.

At the same time, start building a support group of friends who have young children. If you can't find such people, start your own group by hanging a notice in your doctor's waiting room. Or introduce yourself to the people in your childbirth-preparation class. After the birth, you'll want to have friends with babies the same age so you can share experiences, discuss concerns and trade advice.

hidden health risks for working women

>>> **WORKING WOMEN FACE A NUMBER OF CHALLENGES** during pregnancy: scheduling time to see the obstetrician and coping with discomfort on the job, to name a few. But the biggest issue—one that many women aren't even aware of—may be workplace health hazards that could endanger their babies.

According to occupational-health experts, the vast majority of jobs probably are safe for a pregnant woman. However, these experts also note that little is actually known about reproductive hazards in the workplace. They therefore recommend that all women of childbearing age learn as much as possible about potential risks on the job. And the sooner, the better: Whether a woman or her baby is harmed depends on how much of a hazard each is exposed to and when. For instance, babies are vulnerable to environmental exposures as early as the first few weeks after conception.

"For many chemicals, we know what is a safe level for adults to be exposed to. But what may be safe for the adult may not be safe for the developing fetus," says Gideon Koren, M.D., director of the Motherisk Program at the University of Toronto. "Women should be aware of what's around them and seek counseling about potential hazards."

workplace threats

Studies leave little doubt that some types of exposures will harm a developing baby. Organic solvents, for example, are found in many products such as paint and thinners and have been shown to cause miscarriage and birth defects, says Koren, who conducted one such study in 1999. Lead is another substance that is found in many industries, and while it may not be a threat to adults, it poses a risk to developing fetuses. Exposure to a compound called ethylene glycol ether, used in electronics and semiconductor plants, is linked to a higher rate of miscarriage. And carbon monoxide, produced wherever there is combustion, is a known threat to pregnant women and developing babies.

Another potentially dangerous area is in various health care settings. A common virus called cytomegalovirus, which causes mild infections in adults, can be transmitted from a mother to her fetus and cause birth defects. Women in hospitals and clinics also should avoid exposure to ionizing radiation from X-ray and gamma ray machines. (Pregnant women also need to check whether protective gear—like the gloves and masks that health care workers use—fits them properly, since a lot of the gear is made for men.)

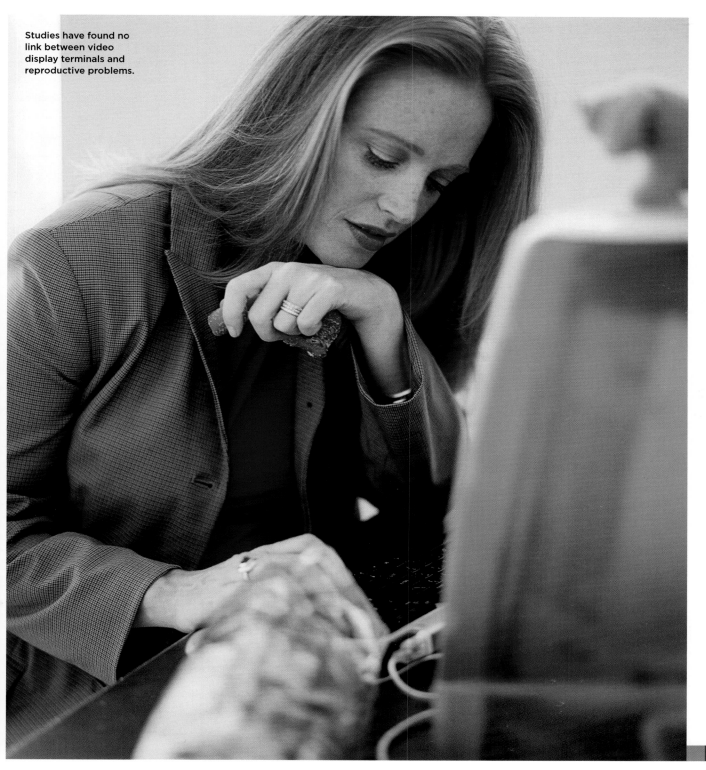

Studies have found no link between video display terminals and reproductive problems.

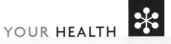
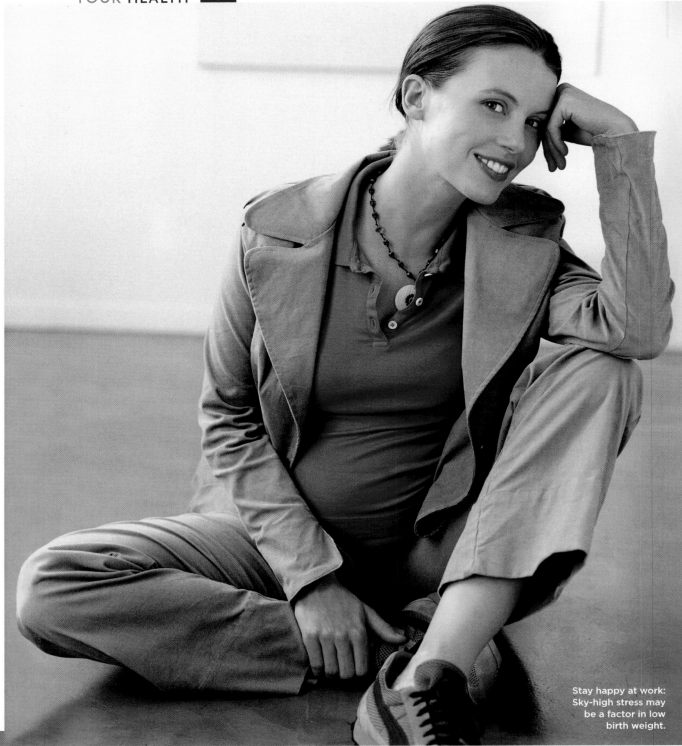

Stay happy at work: Sky-high stress may be a factor in low birth weight.

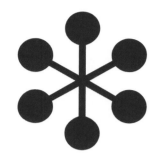

the stress factor

Reproductive-health hazards aren't always chemical in nature. They can also be physical, such as excessive noise, heat, vibration and the exertion required to do a job. For example, a pregnant employee who stands in place for too long or lifts too heavy a load can suffer a cumulative type of stress that increases her risk of developing complications, Koren says.

Peggy Esche thought pregnancy at her desk job at a "family-friendly" company in Wisconsin would be manageable. She was wrong. Long hours of sitting aggravated an inflamed nerve in her back, and swelling in her feet left her unable to wear shoes.

But the real problem was that Esche's stress level soared when strategies to cope with her physical ailments annoyed her employer. Breaks to walk around provoked criticism, and her plea for a more ergonomic workstation was ignored. "I had to find a box from the supply area to prop up my feet to reduce the swelling," she says. "They said they couldn't do anything for me but adjust my chair."

Physical and mental stress are two of the most common health hazards to pregnant women, according to Regina Kenen, M.P.H., author of *Reproductive Hazards in the Workplace* (Haworth Press, 1992). "There should be more slack, more breaks, more flexibility in your work schedule, a comfortable place to sit down, a refrigerator to store healthy food, and good air," she says.

If you encounter resistance, know that you have rights, says Ellen Bravo, national director of 9to5, National Association of Working Women. The federal Pregnancy Discrimination Act offers job protection, as does the Occupational Health and Safety Act and the Family and Medical Leave Act. (Discover how the law protects you: visit *www.9to5.org*.)

"The law protects your rights, but pregnancy is a vulnerable time," Bravo says. "It's when you are least able to muster your resources. Everyone in the workplace, including men, has to work on behalf of all workers."

Workplace stress can contribute to fatigue, headaches and back pain, and it can cause you to lose sleep and eat poorly.

NOT TO WORRY

Pregnant women need not worry about the following factors in a work environment:
- **Noise below 85 decibels** Excessive noise can be a threat, but noise within the occupational limit of 85 decibels is considered safe for all workers.
- **Normal use of some chemicals** The following are unlikely to cause harm: ammonia, asbestos, bleach, chlorine, fiberglass, hydrochloric acid, nitric acid, potassium, silica, sodium hydroxide and sulfuric acid.
- **Video display terminals** Studies have found no link to reproductive problems.

testing 1-2-3

>>> **IT GOES WITH THE TERRITORY: When you're pregnant, you can't help but worry about the health of your baby. Fortunately, there's a host of prenatal tests that can help ease your fears and make even a healthy pregnancy less stressful. Following is a rundown of the tests you're most likely to undergo.**

AMNIOCENTESIS

who needs it and when: Women with a history of birth defects or who will be over 35 at term (or possibly if abnormal maternal serum alpha-fetoprotein results are found); at 15–20 weeks.

what it is: A needle is inserted through the abdomen and into the uterus; a sample of amniotic fluid is withdrawn to test for chromosomal and genetic birth defects such as Down syndrome and spina bifida. Accuracy rate is 99.4 percent.

harm to fetus: Slightly increased risk of miscarriage (1 in 200–400).

follow-up: Depends on findings; genetic counseling may be advised if an abnormality is found.

BLOOD PRESSURE

who needs it and when: All women; at every visit.

what it is: Blood pressure is measured. A sudden rise can signal complications.

harm to fetus: None.

follow-up: If high, additional testing may be needed.

BLOOD SUGAR

who needs it and when: Most women; at 24–28 weeks or when glucose is found in the urine.

what it is: A blood sample, drawn after the mother drinks a sugary mixture, can reveal glucose level in the blood that may indicate gestational diabetes.

harm to fetus: None.

follow-up: If level is high, a change in diet and/or insulin treatment may be prescribed.

BLOOD TYPE AND RH FACTOR

who needs it and when: All pregnant women; at first visit.

what it is: A blood sample is drawn and examined to learn mother's blood type and whether she is Rh-negative.

harm to fetus: None.

follow-up: If Rh-negative, Rh immune globulin is given at 28 weeks.

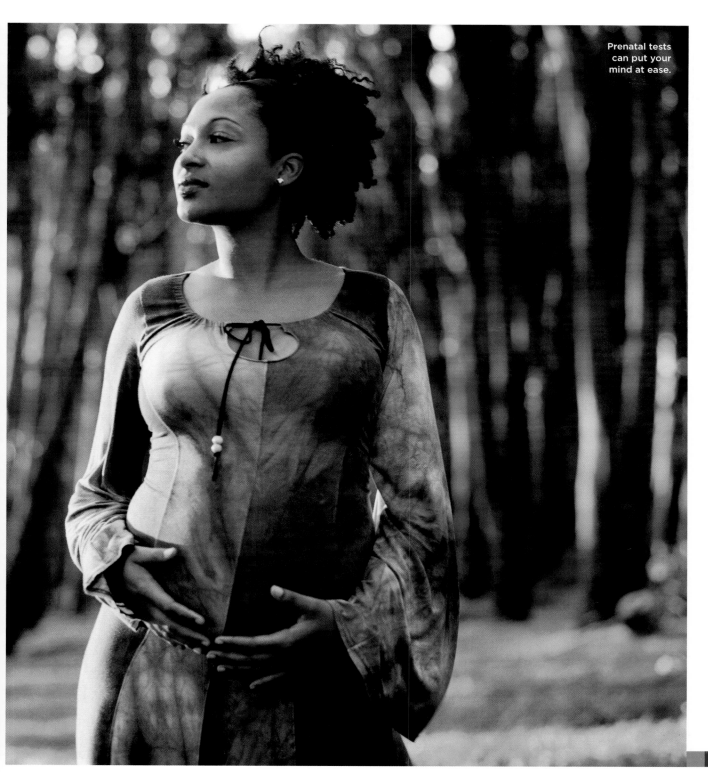

Prenatal tests can put your mind at ease.

CHORIONIC VILLUS SAMPLING

who needs it and when: Women with a history of birth defects or who will be over 35 at term; at 10–12 weeks.

what it is: A needle is inserted through the abdomen and uterus or a catheter is inserted through the vagina and cervix to sample the outer fetal membrane. Chromosomal or genetic birth defects such as Down syndrome or spina bifida can be identified. Accuracy rate is about 98 percent.

harm to fetus: Slightly increased risk of miscarriage (1 in 100–200) and damage to fetus.

follow-up: Depends on findings; genetic counseling may be advised.

CYSTIC FIBROSIS SCREENING

who needs it and when: Women of certain races and ethnicities who are at risk for carrying the disease; early in pregnancy.

what it is: A blood (or, occasionally, saliva) sample is drawn and examined to determine whether mother is a carrier.

harm to fetus: None.

follow-up: If mother is a carrier, the father may be tested; both may be referred for genetic counseling.

GROUP B STREP

who needs it and when: All women; at 35–37 weeks.

what it is: Vagina and perineum are swabbed and sample is examined for presence of potentially deadly bacteria that can be passed to baby at birth.

harm to fetus: None.

follow-up: Antibiotics are given during labor if bacteria are found.

HEMATOCRIT/HEMOGLOBIN

who needs it and when: All women; early in pregnancy and at 32–36 weeks.

what it is: A blood sample is drawn and examined for indication of anemia.

harm to fetus: None.

follow-up: If anemic, extra iron will be prescribed.

MATERNAL SERUM ALPHA-FETOPROTEIN

who needs it and when: All women; at 15–20 weeks.

what it is: Blood is drawn and examined for alpha-fetoprotein, a substance produced by the fetus. Abnormal levels can indicate neural-tube defects, Down syndrome or a multiple pregnancy.

harm to fetus: None.

follow-up: If abnormal levels are found, ultrasound and/or amniocentesis may be suggested to rule out defects or chromosomal errors.

PAP SMEAR/GONORRHEA CULTURE

who needs it and when: Women who have not had a recent Pap smear or who are at risk for having gonorrhea; at first visit.

what it is: Cervical/vaginal secretions are examined for preexisting medical conditions such as cervical cancer and vaginal infections.

harm to fetus: None.

follow-up: Depends on findings.

SCREENING FOR ILLNESSES (HIV, HEPATITIS B, ETC.)

who needs it and when: All women; early in pregnancy. Repeated if mother is exposed to an illness.

what it is: A blood sample is drawn and examined to learn whether mother has been exposed to a disease or illness.

harm to fetus: None.

follow-up: Mother is treated to prevent transmission to fetus at birth.

ULTRASOUND

who needs it and when: Performed as needed to gauge due date or gestational age. Also used during amniocentesis and chorionic villus sampling.

what it is: A device placed on the abdomen or inserted into the vagina creates an image of the fetus. Age and position of fetus, growth rate, placement of placenta and visible defects can all be determined.

harm to fetus: None.

follow-up: Depends on findings; may indicate need for further testing.

URINALYSIS

who needs it and when: All women; at every visit.

what it is: A urine sample is collected and examined. Protein can signal preeclampsia; glucose can signal gestational diabetes.

harm to fetus: None.

follow-up: High levels of protein or glucose require further testing (see blood-sugar test, at left).

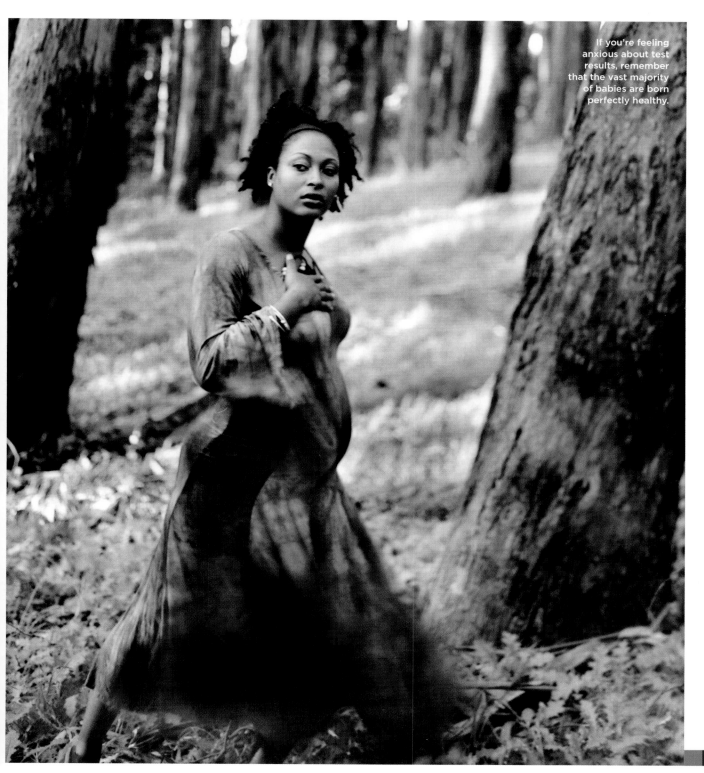

If you're feeling anxious about test results, remember that the vast majority of babies are born perfectly healthy.

Q & A

>>>ANSWERS to questions about your physical and emotional health—and that of your baby.

Q I've heard that Bendectin, the morning-sickness medication that was removed from the market, may be coming back. Is it now considered safe?

A Bendectin was first marketed in the United States in 1956. In 1983, because of numerous lawsuits claiming that the drug caused birth defects, its producer, Merrell Dow Pharmaceuticals, voluntarily withdrew Bendectin from the market. After reviewing 30 years of research, however, experts now believe that Bendectin poses no detectable risk of birth defects. The medication was and is safe to use, and many women who suffer from nausea and resultant dehydration may want to take it to relieve symptoms.

Some doctors treat morning sickness by prescribing the active ingredients in Bendectin—pyroxidene (vitamin B₆) and doxylamine succinate (an antihistamine)— both of which are available over the counter. A Canadian company, Duchesnay Inc., is making a Bendectin-like drug called Diclectin and is negotiating with the U.S. Food and Drug Administration to market a new drug containing the same active ingredients as Bendectin.

Q I'm four months pregnant, and my husband and I want to take our older son to an amusement park. Is it safe for me to go on the rides?

A No. You should stay off all rides with rapid or jerky motions, as the sudden shifting of your baby from one side of the uterus to the other could cause damage to the placenta. You also shouldn't stand in line for a long time, as you put yourself at risk for swollen ankles and blood clots in your legs. So let your husband take your son on the exciting rides as you wave from the sidelines.

Q I'm in my second trimester, and my libido is almost nonexistent. My husband's unhappy and I'm confused. What's going on?

A One of the most common reasons for decreased interest in sex on the part of either a pregnant woman or father-to-be is fear that intercourse will hurt the baby. We're always happy when we get a chance to reassure you that with rare exceptions, you can enjoy sex throughout pregnancy. Natural lubrication shouldn't be a problem, and orgasms are perfectly safe.

Hormones can affect your sex drive, too. Pregnancy triggers constant high levels of estrogen and progesterone, both of which suppress the production of testosterone, a vital hormone where libido is concerned. Fatigue can also be a factor for many women, particularly after a long workday. You might be more responsive after a Saturday afternoon nap.

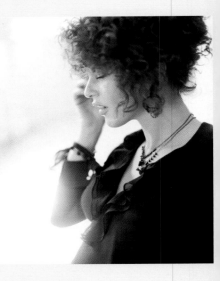

Q I'm 28 years old and have had migraine headaches since I was 20. Now that I'm six weeks pregnant, how can I safely treat them?

A First, avoid dietary triggers such as alcohol, aged cheeses, aspartame (an artificial sweetener) and nitrates (preservatives in bacon, sausage and lunchmeats). Environmental triggers include strong odors such as perfumes and cleaning products.

A soothing compress over the eyes, resting in a dark room or acetaminophen may help minimize symptoms. If your migraine is incapacitating, your doctor may prescribe Fioricet, a non-narcotic sedative. While the prescription drug sumatriptan (Imitrex) is effective in treating migraines, we recommend against its use, particularly in the first trimester—a critical time for embryologic development—as not enough research has been done on it.

Some evidence shows that a sudden decrease in caffeine consumption may be a factor, so if you've abruptly cut out coffee, your migraines may subside after your body adjusts to the change.

Q My doctor wants to screen me for gestational diabetes in my first trimester because my mother developed is Type II diabetes in her 40s. I'm 28—is this test necessary?

A Yes. Your overall health will undoubtedly benefit you and your baby, but since your history includes a first-degree relative who has diabetes, you are at higher risk of developing gestational diabetes. Testing you in the first trimester rather than the third—the standard for women without risk factors—is important.

The test is simple: You'll be asked to drink a 50-gram glucose mixture, and your blood glucose will be measured one hour later. Should your blood glucose indicate gestational diabetes, additional testing will be necessary. If your doctor does find that you have the condition, it can be managed without harm to you or your baby, and it will likely subside after delivery.

Gestational diabetes increases a woman's risk of developing type II diabetes in subsequent pregnancies, or later in life for both mother and baby, so identifying this condition is important.

Q Why is constipation a problem during pregnancy?

A The body's increased production of progesterone, which relaxes the smooth muscles of the uterine wall, intestinal wall and stomach makes digestion sluggish. Also the body tends to become underhydrated as it adjusts to an increasing blood volume. To help prevent constipation, remember to drink at least eight glasses of water every day, consume more fiber and exercise.

Q I'm five months pregnant and have been experiencing a crampy pain on either side of my belly when I get out of bed. Is this normal?

A Yes. You are describing round-ligament pain, which commonly begins around the fourth or fifth month of pregnancy as ligaments stretch to support your increasingly heavy uterus. Many women report a sharp or crampy pain on either side of the abdomen midway between the hip and the bellybutton when getting out of bed, standing up from a seated position or just at random times. The pain usually subsides in a matter of minutes and is nothing to worry about.

You should, however, contact your doctor if you experience severe abdominal pain or recurrent diarrhea or nausea, as these could be symptoms of appendicitis or some other medical problem.

Q I've given up smoking and am planning to get pregnant. Would I put my baby at risk if I become pregnant while using a nicotine patch?

A First off, congrats on quitting. The hazards of tobacco use during pregnancy—including low birth weight and preterm labor—are well-established.

There has not been a great deal of research done about the safety of nicotine-replacement products in pregnant women. Most physicians, however, vigorously recommend that smoking-cessation products such as patches and gum be discontinued during pregnancy. Knowing that you are making a significant, positive impact on your baby's health is the greatest possible incentive to stop using the nicotine patch before conceiving.

Q I know air travel is out late in pregnancy, but I'm in my first trimester and fly occasionally for business. Do I need to stop now?

A Probably not. One concern with air travel is exposure to solar radiation, as excessive amounts of any type of radiation may put a fetus at increased risk for childhood cancers. However, the experts state that such risks from "casual" air travel are negligible.

The National Council on Radiation Protection and Measurements recommends that a pregnant woman receive no more than 1 millisievert of radiation exposure during her pregnancy. One round-trip, cross-country flight delivers 6 percent of that; a round-trip New York-Tokyo flight constitutes 15 percent. Occasional travel is therefore within the safe range of exposure. Pregnant women who travel frequently or work on airplanes may need to modify their schedules. For a per-trip radiation calculator, visit *http://jag.cami.jccbi. gov/cariprofile.asp.*

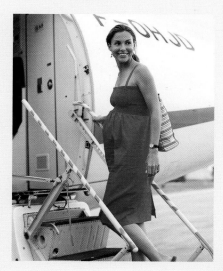

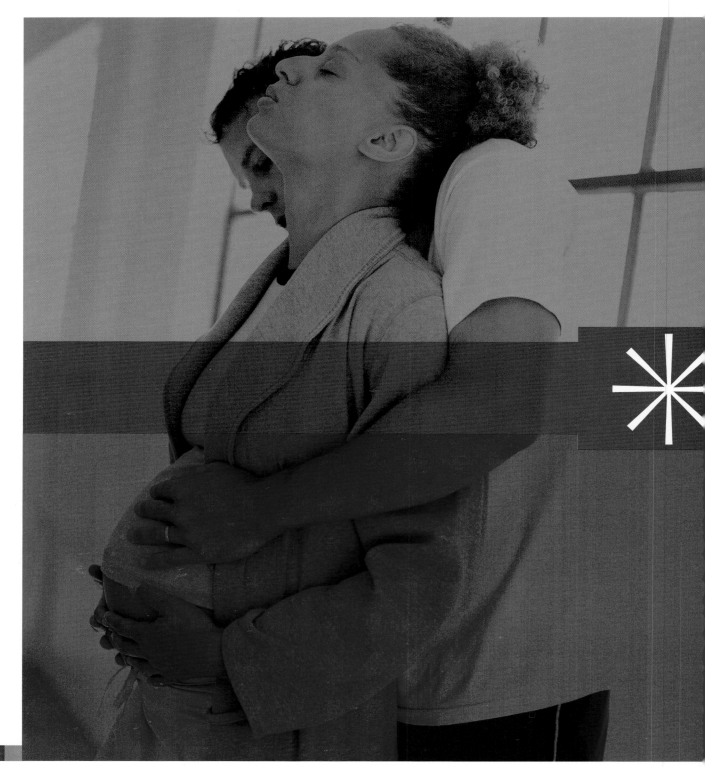

your labor and delivery

>>> FROM THE MOMENT you discover you're pregnant, decisions await you. Fortunately, many of them, such as what color to paint the nursery and whether to use disposable diapers, are not life-changing. But the big-picture decisions—like where your baby will be born, who will deliver her and whether you should schedule the birth—can have a profound impact on your pregnancy and delivery, often making the difference between a joyous experience you can't wait to repeat and a traumatic one you'd rather forget.

We're here to help, with information to guide you through these and other choices, such as whether to get an epidural or to try for a vaginal birth after having a Cesarean. We also provide lots of practical advice, including surprising tips for an easier labor.

Finally, though no two labor and delivery experiences are exactly alike, our outline of what happens in the final hours of pregnancy can help you prepare for the most exciting day of your life: your baby's birth day. Wherever you are in your journey toward motherhood, be sure to keep this guide handy.

in this chapter:
* where will you have your baby?
* who will deliver?
* childbirth education
* pain relief
* natural birth
* scheduling delivery
* labor anxiety
* C-sections
* fetal distress
* first signs of labor
* what happens during delivery
* Q & A

your guide to giving birth

>>> **REMEMBER THAT THE BEST-LAID DELIVERY PLANS are** just that—plans. Naturally, you'll need to decide where you'll have your baby and who will deliver her. And in today's high-tech world, *how* you'll deliver and even *when* can be up to you as well—baby willing, of course. After reading this chapter, make a wish list and show it to your doctor to see if what you want is possible. Just be sure to go into labor with a very open mind!

where will you have your baby?

at the hospital

If you have pregnancy complications or risk factors for a C-section, prefer an obstetrician to a midwife or want to receive labor-induction and/or pain medication, a hospital birth is for you. If your insurance lets you choose, here's a checklist of what to look for. Keep in mind that few hospitals meet all these criteria.

> An obstetrician is on the premises at all times.
> The hospital's maternal mortality rate is at or below 0.01 percent.
> There is a neonatal intensive-care unit of at least level II (level III is best).
> The primary C-section rate is at or below the national average of 26 percent.
> The hospital does not limit when you can receive pain medication.
> The hospital has a lactation consultant on staff.
> Midwives are allowed to deliver babies, and doula services are permitted.
> The same nurses care for you throughout labor, delivery and recovery.
> During labor, women are allowed to walk around and use private bathtubs or showers.
> Women can give birth in rooms specifically geared for labor/delivery and recovery.
> There is a place for the father to sleep overnight.
> The baby can stay in your room with you.
> Friends and relatives besides the father are allowed to attend the birth.
> Water births, videotaping of births and massage services are permitted and/or available.
> Classes on infant care, breastfeeding, sibling relationships and the like are offered.

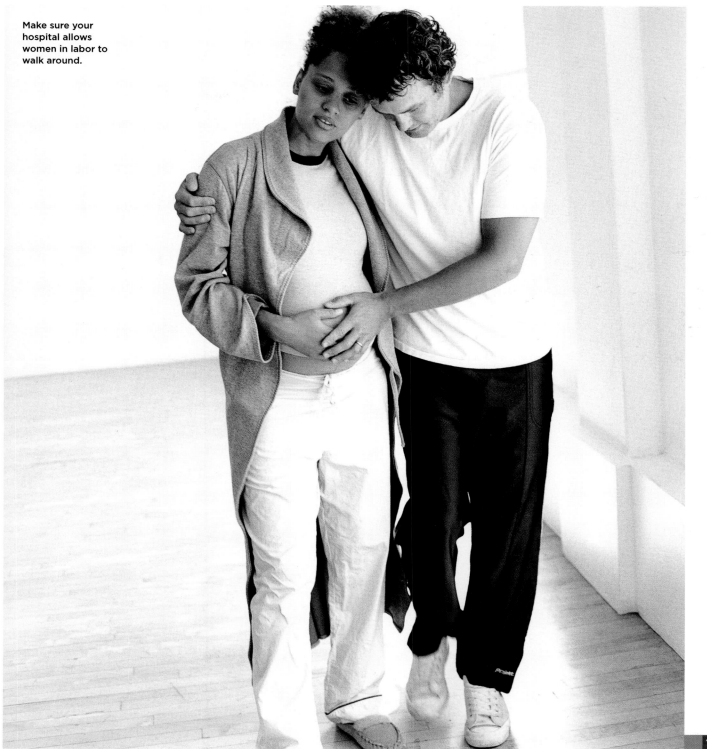

Make sure your hospital allows women in labor to walk around.

at the birth center

Freestanding (nonhospital) birth centers offer women with uncomplicated pregnancies who want a natural delivery a less high-tech, more homelike alternative to hospitals. Babies generally are delivered by midwives, and women are allowed to give birth in the position that's most comfortable for them. "Birth centers don't offer epidurals or [the labor-induction drug] Pitocin, and they only take low-risk patients," says Kate Bauer, executive director of the National Association of Childbearing Centers, based in Perkiomenville, Pa. "What they do offer is education-intensive care from the prenatal period through six weeks postpartum."

According to a recent study in the *American Journal of Public Health,* most women who plan to give birth at freestanding birth centers end up succeeding, with fewer C-sections and medical interventions. While about 15 percent of women are transferred to a hospital, this is usually because of failure to progress, Bauer says. "Most of these women go on to give birth vaginally," she adds. Bauer suggests looking for a birth center with the following features:

> The staff are advocates for natural childbirth and breastfeeding.

> An extensive support system is in place.

> The baby can stay in the room with you.

> The center is accredited by the Commission for the Accreditation of Birth Centers.

Today, an increasing number of hospitals have on-site birth centers. In these homey, comfortable rooms, your baby will stay with you and, because it will be assumed that you are breastfeeding, won't be given a bottle. "Some hospitals have adopted certain philosophies of our freestanding birth centers, and we think that's great," Bauer says. For more information, go to *www.birthcenters.org.*

at home

Most women who want a home birth believe that having a baby is a natural process requiring little medical intervention. Many also want more control and attention than they might get in a hospital or even a birth center. Here's what you should know:

> Home birth isn't for everyone. Medical conditions that make a hospital the safer choice include high blood pressure, diabetes, severe anemia, preterm labor, unexplained vaginal bleeding, carrying multiples, a pregnancy that goes beyond 42 weeks or a baby in the breech position.

> European studies show that for a healthy woman with a low-risk pregnancy, home birth can be a safe option. However, the American College of Obstetricians and Gynecologists maintains that the hospital is the safest place to give birth. For example, in about 1 percent of pregnancies, the placenta separates from the wall of the uterus; such an emergency requires immediate medical intervention that's not possible at home.

> Most home births are attended by midwives. But you should enlist an OB-GYN as a medical backup (many midwives will refer) and find a pediatrician who'll see the baby within 48 hours.

> You should live no more than 30 minutes from a hospital. Transfer to a hospital occurs in one out of 10 planned home births attended by certified nurse-midwives.

> You'll be giving up some forms of medical assistance. "You're making a commitment to a natural childbirth," says Alice Bailes, former chairwoman of the home-birth committee of the American College of Nurse-Midwives. That means no drugs to speed labor and no epidural for pain.

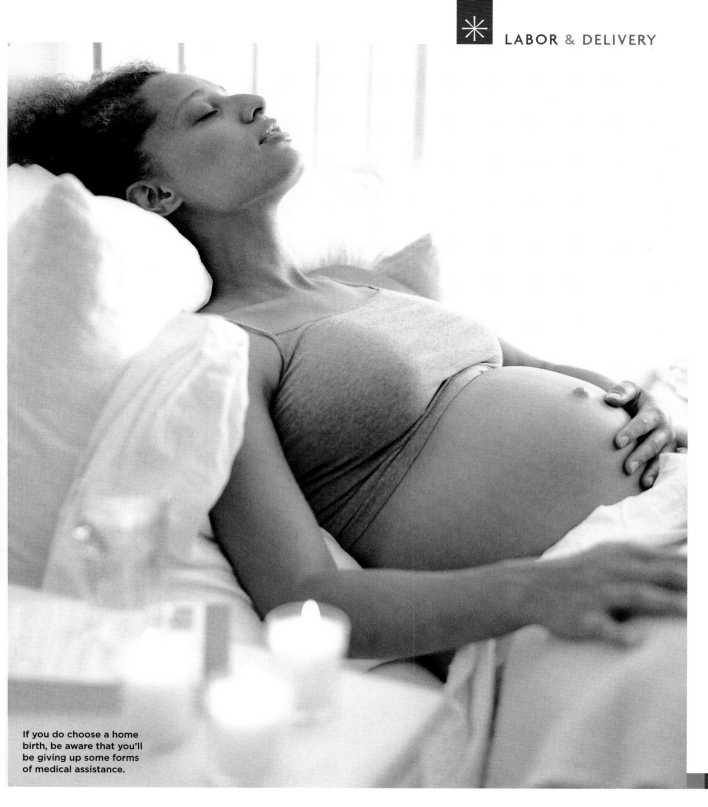

If you do choose a home birth, be aware that you'll be giving up some forms of medical assistance.

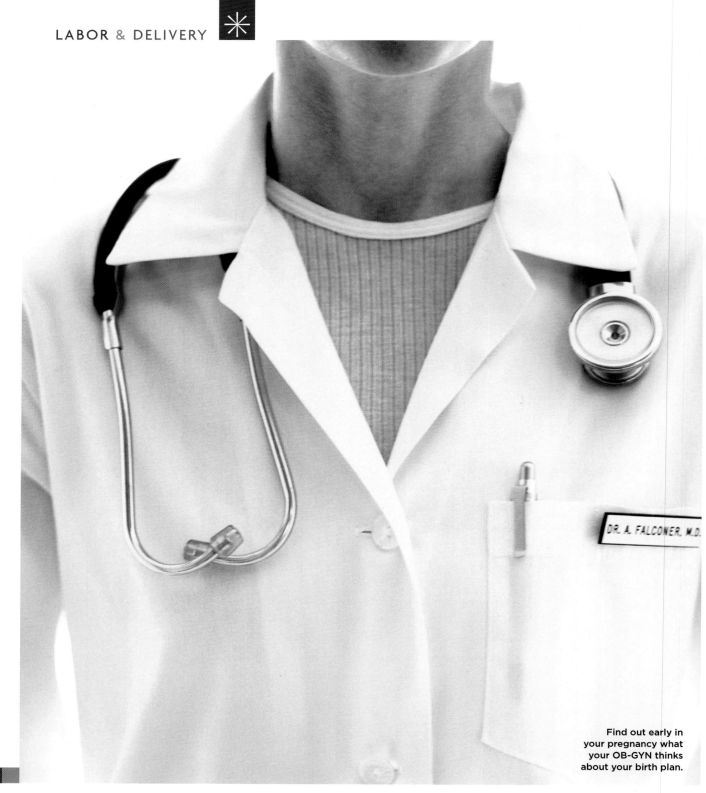

DR. A. FALCONER, M.D.

Find out early in
your pregnancy what
your OB-GYN thinks
about your birth plan.

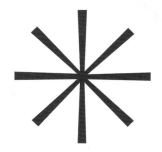

Midwives have a philosophy of care that encourages the woman to actively participate. So feel free to discuss with her any and all options.

who will deliver your baby?

Take some time to consider who you'd like to deliver your baby. The two main options are an obstetrician or a midwife. When making the doctor-versus-midwife decision, here are some of the things you may get (and give up) with each:

THE OBSTETRICIAN

Pros: Can handle high-risk pregnancies and delivery emergencies; can administer or order pain-relief drugs; has a support staff.
Cons: Typically spends less time during prenatal appointments and labor; consistency of care may be lacking if the doctor is part of a large medical group; your doctor may not be on call when you're ready to give birth.
For more information: Visit *www.acog.org*.

THE MIDWIFE

Pros: Provides supportive, collaborative care; offers nonmedical pain-relief alternatives; provides information on alternative birthing positions and methods; increases the chance of having an unmedicated delivery and avoiding a Cesarean section.
Cons: Can't handle high-risk pregnancies and some delivery emergencies.
For more information: Visit *www.acnm.org*.

For an extensive list of questions to ask when selecting a caregiver, visit *www.maternity wise.org* and click on "Questions to ask."

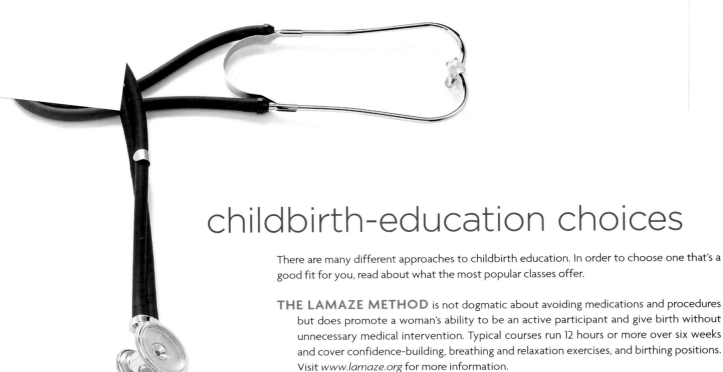

childbirth-education choices

There are many different approaches to childbirth education. In order to choose one that's a good fit for you, read about what the most popular classes offer.

THE LAMAZE METHOD is not dogmatic about avoiding medications and procedures but does promote a woman's ability to be an active participant and give birth without unnecessary medical intervention. Typical courses run 12 hours or more over six weeks and cover confidence-building, breathing and relaxation exercises, and birthing positions. Visit *www.lamaze.org* for more information.

THE BRADLEY METHOD (aka husband-coached childbirth) makes a mission of natural childbirth and claims that 87 percent of graduates who deliver vaginally do so without medication. Courses typically run 30 hours over 12 weeks and cover prenatal nutrition and fitness, muscle awareness and relaxation techniques. Partners coach women through everything from preparatory pelvic tilts to final-stage pushing. For more information, visit *www.bradleybirth.com*.

BIRTHING FROM WITHIN is typically an eight-week course (two classes are postpartum) in which couples explore their hopes and fears about labor and delivery. They learn about the physical processes but also delve into emotional issues such as how they will deal with an unplanned C-section or other unwished-for surprises. Visit *www.birthing fromwithin.com* for details.

BIRTH WORKS promotes the belief that knowing how to give birth is inherent in every woman, thus helping expectant moms to have more trust and faith in their bodies. In classes that typically run 10 weeks, students explore their beliefs and attitudes about childbirth through expression of feelings, sensory visualization and art. See *www.birth works.org* for more information.

HYPBIRTH is an interactive CD and video program that's used in the later stages of pregnancy and during delivery. Designed to teach women self-hypnosis and change their perception of labor, it boasts a success rate of 80 percent to 90 percent unmedicated deliveries. For more details, visit *www.hypbirth.com*.

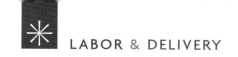

pain-relief options

Knowing your pain-relief choices can help when you're considering natural childbirth versus a medicated delivery. Here's a look at the most common methods.

	CHOICES	WHEN IT IS USED	PROS	CONS
DRUGS	Epidural injection	Anytime during labor, but many doctors wait until it's well under way	Virtually eliminates pain; dosage and timing can be adjusted	Might lengthen labor; can cause fever or headache
	Opioid injection	Throughout labor	Can be given more than once	Not very effective; might make baby sleepy
	Nitrous-oxide inhalation	Continuously or during contractions	Safe and effective; no needles	Can be difficult to time with contractions; not widely available
ALTERNATIVES	Warm bath (1–2 hours)	Best after labor is well under way	Might delay or reduce use of drugs	Effects are temporary; not always available
	Walking	Throughout labor	Can give the mother a sense of control	Not always an option
	Sterile water injection (for back pain)	Throughout labor	Inexpensive; can delay or reduce use of drugs	Slightly painful to administer; pain relief temporary
	Touch and massage	Throughout labor	Can be done by partner or other person	May not alleviate severe pain
	Doula (or other nonmedical labor support)	Throughout labor	No negative side effects	Usually requires advance planning; may not be covered by insurance

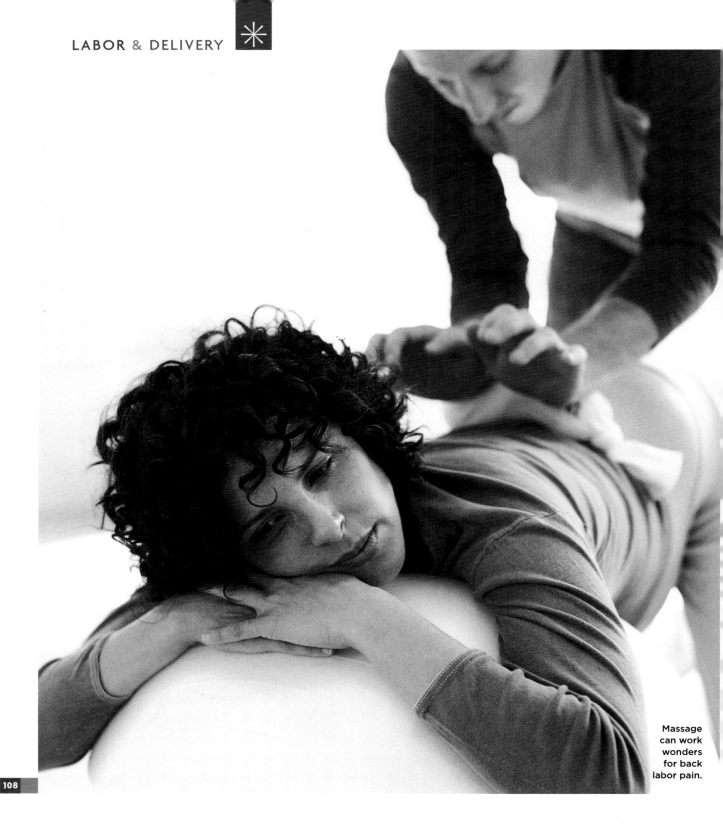

Massage
can work
wonders
for back
labor pain.

6 ways to increase your chances of a natural birth

Though statistics are scarce, some approaches are known, at least anecdotally, to increase the odds of having an unmedicated delivery:

1) Use a midwife Studies show that using a properly trained, licensed midwife rather than an obstetrician can greatly increase your chances for giving birth naturally. The extra attention pays off in less anxiety and pain. For referrals: American College of Nurse-Midwives, *www.midwife.org*.

2) Hire a doula A doula is a woman trained to provide mothers and their families with encouragement and information through late pregnancy, labor and delivery. A review of six studies of more than 2,000 women found that with the continuous support of a trained doula, epidural use decreased by 60 percent, C-sections by 50 percent, drug use for labor induction by 40 percent, forceps use by 40 percent and average length of labor by 25 percent. For referrals and more information: Association of Labor Assistants & Childbirth Educators (ALACE), *www.alace.org*; Doulas of North America (DONA), *www.dona.org*; International Childbirth Education Association (ICEA), *www.icea.org*.

3) Practice self-hypnosis "For a gentle, natural birth, the muscles of your uterus need oxygen-carrying blood," says Marie Mongan, founder of HypnoBirthing, a program that teaches pregnant women self-hypnosis techniques for use during labor (visit *www.hypnobirthing.com* for details). "Fear directs blood away from the uterus, and the result is more pain." The American Society of Clinical Hypnosis reports that for about two-thirds of women who use hypnosis, it is their sole analgesic during labor.

4) Learn perineal massage By relaxing and stretching the area around the vagina during pregnancy, perineal massage may safely help speed delivery, lessening the need for painkillers. Do this for six to eight minutes daily, beginning no earlier than 34 weeks into your pregnancy.

5) Take childbirth ed Several courses focus on unmedicated deliveries. Enroll as early as possible; classes fill up fast, and some, such as Bradley, run 12 weeks, so you need to start them in your second trimester. (For more childbirth education options, see our guide on page 106.)

6) Get into warm water Doing so can naturally facilitate labor and ease pain. You can climb into a tub for a few hours, then get out to have the baby. Or you may decide on a water birth. For information, visit *www.waterbirth.org*.

3 TIPS FOR AN EASIER LABOR

1. Set the mood A dark, quiet environment is ideal, so ask for dim lights and minimal noise.

2. Stuff a sock Bring a tube sock with three tennis balls in it and have your partner or someone else roll them up and down your back to relieve pain.

3. Get on the ball Drape your upper body faceup over a large exercise ball to relieve back pain. Or sit on it with your legs apart to relax the pelvic area.

LABOR ANXIETY

While just about every pregnant woman feels some anxiety about labor and delivery, 6 percent to 10 percent suffer intense fear that manifests itself as nightmares, physical complaints, difficulty concentrating or other symptoms. If left unchecked, fear and its associated stress can contribute to both early and late deliveries, smaller babies and a higher risk for emergency C-section. What's more, frightened women may actually experience more discomfort during childbirth. The good news is that there are ways to reduce your fear of childbirth. Here are five:

1) Track the source Certain experiences can trigger an intense fear of labor, including past abuse or rape; miscarriage or stillbirth; guilt over an abortion; a previous difficult delivery; and exposure to traumatic labor stories.

2) Consider therapy In one study, women with an intense fear of labor who underwent cognitive (talk) therapy had shorter labors and fewer unnecessary C-sections than those who didn't.

3) Tell your doctor Your OB-GYN probably has ideas about how to reduce your anxiety. Also discuss your feelings about medication, episiotomy and similar issues during a prenatal visit.

4) Shut out negative stories Don't watch scary TV shows about childbirth or listen to friends recount the gory details of their labors.

5) Be open-minded about drugs Knowing that effective means of pain relief are available (see page 107) can help lessen your anxiety.

scheduling your delivery

More women are choosing their baby's birth date for a variety of reasons, including fear of the unexpected, work considerations and vacation schedules for school-age children. But scheduling an induction or a first-time C-section isn't without risk—or debate.

Inducing labor with drugs is one way to help ensure that childbirth occurs in a specific 24- to 48-hour period. In 2001, nearly 21 percent of babies were delivered after labor was induced—up from 8 percent in 1989, according to the American College of Obstetricians and Gynecologists (ACOG). This does not mean that inductions are always safe. According to Michael F. Greene, M.D., director of maternal-fetal medicine at Massachusetts General Hospital in Boston, induction increases the chances of a C-section by 50 percent and should only be done when risks of continuing the pregnancy, such as having high blood pressure or being two weeks overdue, exceed the risk posed by inducing labor. "ACOG is against inducing labor just because you want the baby to be a Sagittarius," Greene says.

Induction isn't always successful, either. Hormones such as oxytocin are released when labor starts naturally. But administering Pitocin, the synthetic version of oxytocin, does not guarantee that labor will necessarily begin or progress easily. In fact, if Pitocin is given too aggressively, extremely frequent and intense contractions can result.

Some doctors say that women who are determined to schedule labor are better off planning C-sections instead of inductions. This is because a scheduled Cesarean often is easier on the body than a long, induced labor that may end with an emergency C-section anyway.

Emergency C-sections also are more rushed than planned Cesareans are, thus they increase the possibility of complications. But even a scheduled C-section can require weeks and sometimes months of healing and can carry an increased risk of infection and blood loss. It's not a decision to be made lightly. (See "If You Have a C-Section" on page 113.)

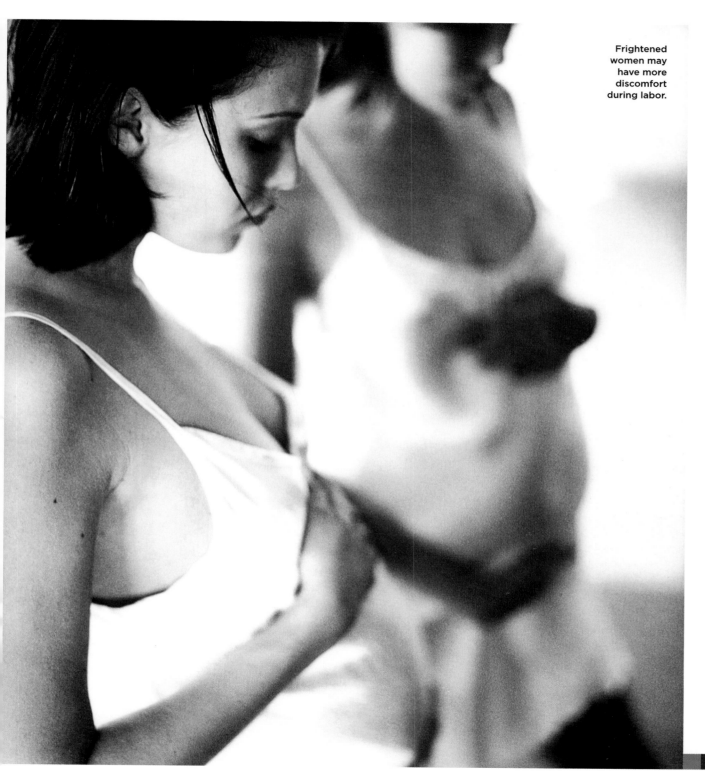

Frightened
women may
have more
discomfort
during labor.

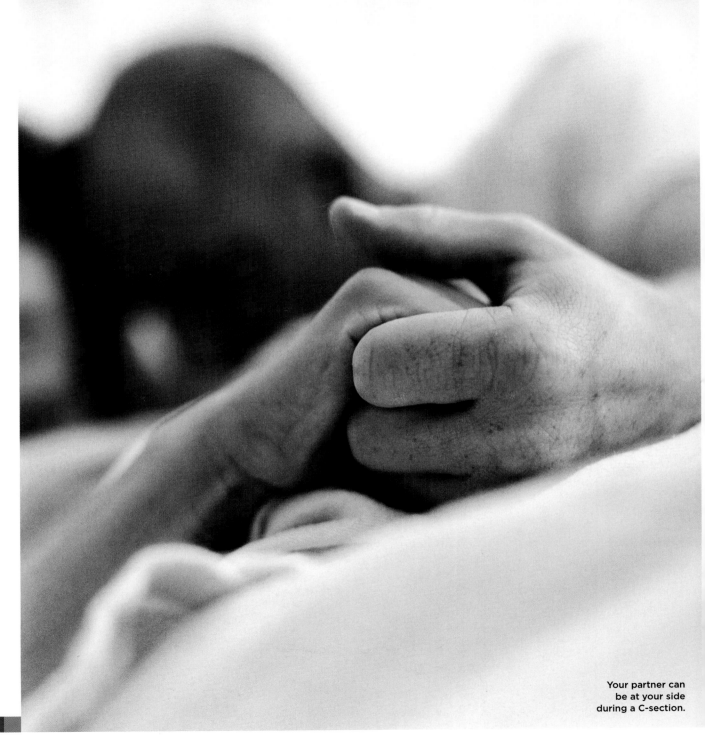

Your partner can
be at your side
during a C-section.

if you have a C-section

Whether or not your C-section is planned, here's generally what you can expect.

- **A nurse will start an IV** containing saline solution and, in some cases, an antibiotic. Unless the C-section is an emergency, the anesthesiologist will administer an epidural so you won't feel anything below your belly button (though you'll be fully awake). Otherwise, you may receive a general anesthetic.

- **Your doctor will drape the area around your belly,** then cut through the skin, muscles, uterus and amniotic sac. "You feel almost nothing—maybe a little pressure and some tugging," says Gloria Bachmann, M.D., chief of the OB-GYN Service at the Robert Wood Johnson University Hospital in New Brunswick, N.J. Minutes later, the doctor will lift the baby out and bring her up to your head for you to see. Then the doctor will remove the placenta and stitch you up. The entire process will take 40 to 90 minutes.

- **Nurses will monitor your blood pressure,** breathing and heart rate in the recovery room. (You might become nauseated and start vomiting at this point; this is normal.) After an hour or so, you'll be moved to your room and reunited with your baby, and you'll probably be able to breastfeed at this time.

- **You'll experience gas pains and pain at the incision site** in the following days and perhaps weeks. Like women who deliver vaginally, you'll need to wear pads for several weeks to absorb the blood-tinged fluid that will flow from your uterus as you recuperate.

fetal distress

Though it has no universally agreed-upon definition, fetal distress is characterized as a slowing ("deceleration") of the baby's heart rate at times during labor when it shouldn't. In many cases, doctors have plenty of time to consider their options, which include vacuum extraction, delivery with forceps or untangling the umbilical cord from around the baby's neck. But when fetal distress occurs suddenly—the uterus is rupturing, for example—doctors have only minutes to get the baby out to avoid brain damage or even death. When this happens, doctors tend to err on the side of caution and do a C-section.

Sometimes babies who are stressed in utero pass their first stool (meconium) while still in the birth canal. If it's inhaled, a lung infection or pneumonia can result. In such cases, the baby's mouth is suctioned as soon as the head is delivered.

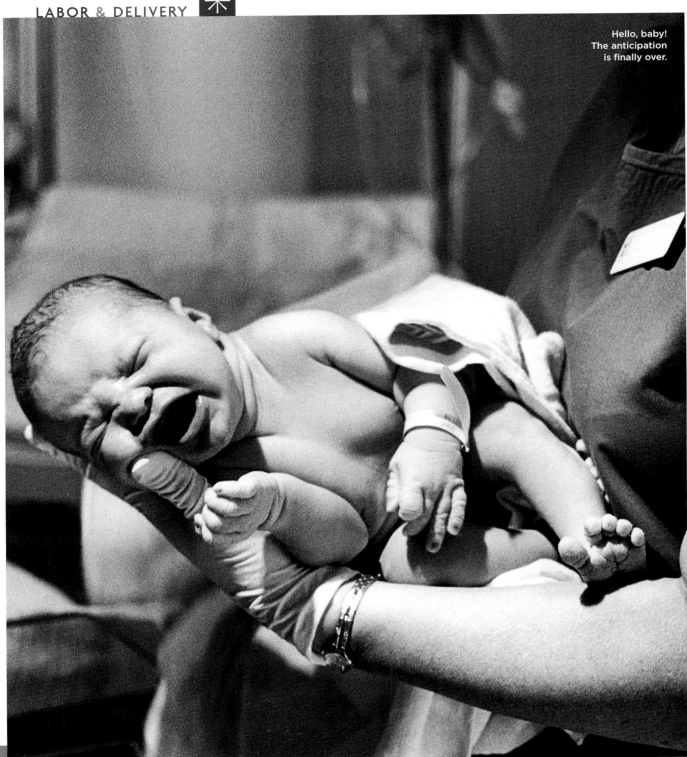

Hello, baby!
The anticipation
is finally over.

what happens during delivery

EARLY LABOR (typically 5 to 8 hours) When contractions begin, your cervix is effacing (thinning) and dilating (opening from 0 to 3 centimeters). On average, it opens about 1 centimeter per hour. Contractions usually are mild at first but build in strength and frequency. Once these start coming every five minutes, most doctors will tell you to go to the hospital.

Generally, the nurses will hook you up to an IV (to prevent dehydration) and to an electronic monitor that measures your baby's heart rate and your uterine contractions. Your doctor or midwife will do an internal exam to check your progress. You may be offered a mild pain reliever such as Demerol or Stadol, and if you want an epidural, it may be started now (though they are typically started later).

ACTIVE LABOR (typically 2 to 8 hours) Your cervix will dilate from 4 to 7 centimeters. Contractions will be stronger, longer and closer together, and the breathing and relaxation exercises you learned in childbirth class will come in handy.

TRANSITION (15 minutes to 1 hour or longer) Your cervix will dilate from 8 to 10 centimeters. "This is the really intense phase of labor," says Joan Edwards, M.N., C.N.S., assistant clinical professor at Texas Women's University in Houston. "It's when women say things like, 'I can't do this anymore!'" Swearing up a storm or becoming angry at your husband (and vowing never to have sex again) are perfectly normal during this time.

PUSHING (a few minutes to 3 hours) When you're dilated 10 centimeters, it's time to push. You feel lots of pressure in the rectal area, as if you're trying to pass a bowel movement. Pushing can be exhausting, but many women find it's a relief to start. "I thought the pushing part was pretty easy, especially since the epidural had just kicked in," says Courtenay Manes Labson of Chevy Chase, Md. "It felt productive, whereas labor prior to that point had felt more reactive. I also think being in good shape physically made pushing more doable." As the baby's head first begins to show, your doctor may perform an episiotomy if she feels it's necessary (see Q & A on page 117).

AFTER THE BABY IS BORN Within 30 minutes you'll be asked to push again to deliver the placenta, which usually comes out easily. If you've had an episiotomy, your doctor will then stitch you up. And you'll get to hold your baby for the first time.

THE SIGNS OF LABOR

Braxton Hicks contractions (aka false labor) These often start three to four weeks or more before delivery. The irregular, mild tightness or cramping lasts a few seconds. Unlike true contractions, these won't get more regular or intense.

Lightening ("dropping") The baby descends into the pelvis as early as two to four weeks before labor. You'll feel pressure on your rectum and may need to urinate more.

Loss of the mucous plug The expulsion of a glob of mucous from the cervix can occur anywhere from one or two weeks to just hours before labor—or not at all. When tinged with blood, it's called "bloody show."

Water breaking The amniotic-fluid sac (aka membranes or "bag of waters") may rupture before labor starts, releasing warm fluid. Call your doctor if you think your water has broken.

Q & A

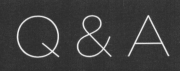

>>> ANSWERS to your questions about labor, birth, C-sections and more

Q I'm a healthy 30-year-old who is pregnant for the first time. What do you think about using a midwife for my labor and delivery?

A The certified nurse-midwives (CNMs) have excellent training in nursing and obstetrics. They also have a sensitive approach to birthing, a deep understanding of pain control and innovative strategies for utilizing the patient's birth coach. CNMs may independently manage labor and delivery for low-risk patients or consult with an obstetrician when needed. Licensing, titles and certification of midwives vary from state to state. Visit the Web site of the American College of Nurse-Midwives at *www.midwife.org* to learn about midwives in your area.

Q Whatever happened to what were once known as "birth plans"?

A Yesterday's pages of written instructions are giving way to wish lists that outline what expectant moms would *like* to happen during labor. At one time, notations may have instructed health care givers to forgo things like fetal monitoring, IVs with drugs and epidurals. Today's more prevalent wish-list guidelines may ask for sporadic fetal monitoring; a heparin lock (a needle is inserted in case you need an IV, but is not attached to anything); and "going with the flow" before opting for an epidural.

Q What exactly are the benefits to "laboring down"?

A Laboring down (aka waiting to push) may be, in some cases, a wise option. Women who receive epidurals may have less complicated deliveries if their doctors ask them to delay pushing until after the cervix is completely dilated to 10 centimeters. Here's why: Waiting a few hours before pushing allows the continuing contractions to help propel the baby into the pelvis. This technique can prolong labor by three hours or more.

Studies have been inconclusive as to whether women who labor down need fewer C-sections or forceps deliveries, and until more research is conducted, there is no way to know whether waiting to push will benefit all or even most women. Some doctors do believe, however, that a woman whose baby is in a posterior position is the most likely to benefit.

Q Last month, my best friend had her labor induced and gave birth to a 10-pound baby boy. Is labor always induced when a baby is that large?

A No. The induction of labor due only to a baby's size, or a desire to time delivery to make it convenient for the doctor or patient, is not appropriate, according to many obstetric standards. Our personal belief is that induction should only be considered when it supports the safety of the mother and the baby.

There are cases when induction is appropriate, however. The American College of Obstetricians and Gynecologists (ACOG) has reported that the rate of labor induction increased from 9.5 percent to 19.4 percent between 1990 and 1998. This increase represents, in part, our better understanding of at-risk near-term pregnancies, which in turn has increased our ability to induce based on concrete medical considerations. A woman should not be a candidate for induction of labor due to the size of her baby unless her cervix is "favorable," or ready to be responsive to the agents used to induce labor.

Q My last baby was delivered by Cesarean section. This time I'd like to try for a vaginal delivery. What, if any, are the risks with a VBAC?

A In the early '90s, when many women learned they could safely deliver vaginally after a prior C-section, the rate of VBACs (vaginal birth after C-section) rose steadily—by 50 percent—until 1997. Then came reports that VBAC increased the risk of uterine rupture, an emergency situation that's potentially deadly for both mother and baby. The VBAC rate plummeted from 28.3 percent in 1996 to just 12.7 percent in 2002. Research later reported in *The New England Journal of Medicine* found that the risk for uterine rupture was largely linked to certain induction drugs.

Today, many doctors say VBAC is safe, as long as labor is not induced. But the most important precaution is choosing a hospital that is prepared to handle VBAC emergencies. Before attempting a VBAC, consult with your doctor; she'll take into consideration why you had the prior C-section, the type of incision you had and whether you had a fever afterward.

Q Are episiotomies still a routine procedure at most hospitals?

A An episiotomy is an incision that widens the vaginal opening so the baby's head can pass through more easily. For decades, obstetricians routinely performed episiotomies, believing an incision would prevent serious tears and pelvic-floor muscle damage, which can contribute to incontinence. But new

research has found that nearly 8 percent of women who have episiotomies develop serious tears, compared with 3.6 percent of women who don't have them, and that the procedure may increase, not reduce, damage to pelvic-floor muscles.

ACOG denounced routine episiotomies in 2000, but some doctors continue to perform them needlessly. An episiotomy is warranted when a forceps or vacuum-suction delivery is needed, or when a baby is very large or needs to be delivered quickly. Ask your doctor what her episiotomy rate is and what factors have prompted her to perform them.

Q I'm six months pregnant. My best friend just had a baby and said delivery of the placenta was painful. Is this always the case?

A This is often the case. Delivery of the placenta is the final stage of childbirth; 95 percent of the time, it occurs within about 15 minutes of the baby's birth. The uterus still needs to work after delivering the baby, first expelling the placenta (which usually weighs about 1 pound) and then pushing it through the birth canal. So, yes, you may experience some pain with these contractions. But that pain is usually secondary to overwhelming relief: Your baby has finally arrived!

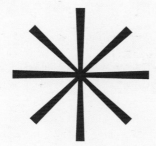

Though you may have some pain when the placenta is delivered, it's usually secondary to overwhelming relief: Your baby has finally arrived!

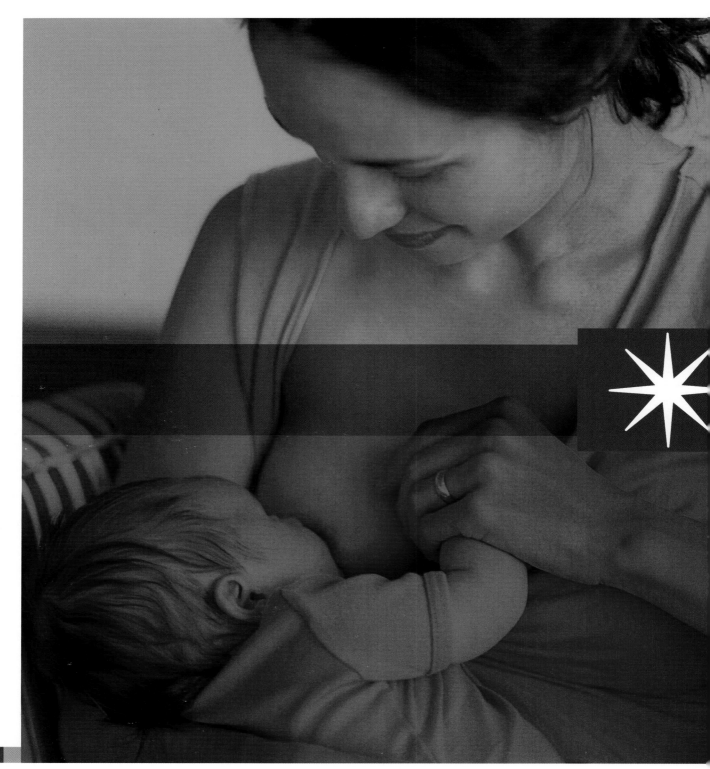

breastfeeding basics

Nursing is a learned skill. Here are the best strategies for success.

>>> IF SOMEONE TOLD YOU there's an elixir that could help protect your new baby from bronchitis, ear infections, pneumonia, diarrhea and urinary tract infections, would you want to know more? If you knew that the effects of this concoction would last into your child's teenage years, reducing his risk for diabetes, allergies and high blood pressure, would you just have to have it? If the same potion might boost his IQ, wouldn't you rush out to find it?

As you most likely know, this power-packed product is your very own breast milk. While you might believe it's premature to start thinking about breastfeeding when you're still months away from delivery, studies show that making a commitment now will boost your chances of successful breastfeeding later. On the following pages, discover the strategies that will help you provide your newborn with nature's best possible nutrition.

in this chapter:
* ✳ enlist your partner's help
* ✳ take a class
* ✳ "room in"
* ✳ put baby to your breast
* ✳ get the right latch
* ✳ seek support
* ✳ set small goals
* ✳ the laundry can wait
* ✳ Q & A

breastfeeding made easy

>>> **MANY WOMEN APPROACH BREASTFEEDING** with an all-or-nothing attitude, assuming that they'll breastfeed exclusively and that it will be an effortless, even blissful experience. After all, why shouldn't something so natural be easy? The good news is, for many women, nursing is trouble-free. But as any lactation consultant, doctor or girlfriend will tell you, breastfeeding also is a learned art, one that requires education, practice and plenty of support. With that in mind, we asked several leading lactation consultants to give us their best breastfeeding tips. Here are the eight things they believe every nursing mom should know and do.

1. Enlist your partner's help early on

Breastfeeding may be something only you can do for your baby, but it's much easier to accomplish when you have the full support of your husband or partner. What can he do to help? Plenty. During pregnancy, he can reinforce your committment to nurse. In those overwhelming first weeks after you give birth, when your primary goals are to rest, care for your baby and establish a good milk supply, he can prepare the meals, take over errands and household chores, deal with phone calls and visitors, and make sure that you're eating and drinking enough. If you're feeling exhausted and discouraged early on, your partner's encouragement and positive attitude may make all the difference.

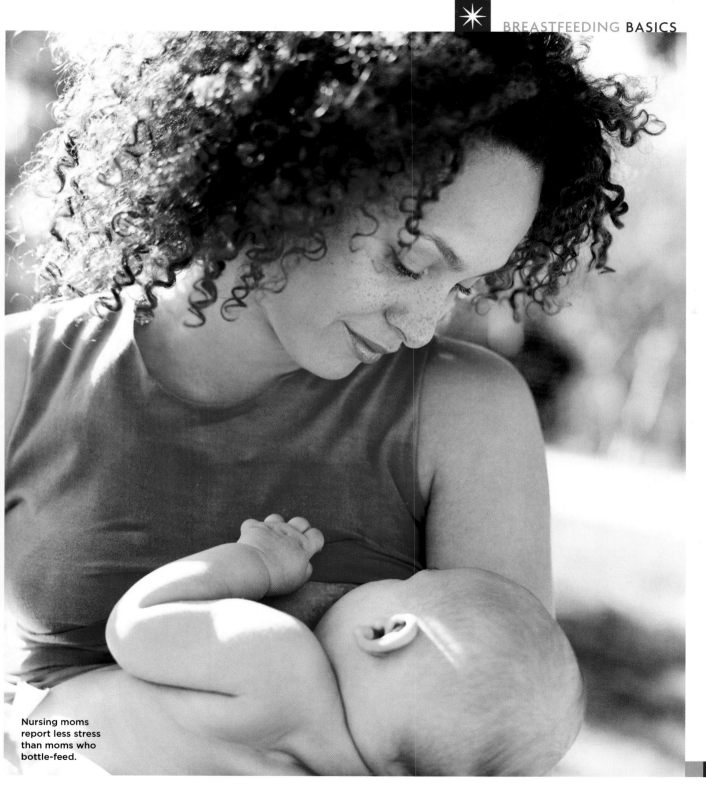

Nursing moms
report less stress
than moms who
bottle-feed.

2. Take a breastfeeding class

The more you know beforehand, the more prepared you'll feel when your baby arrives. So in addition to reading and talking to other women, take a class on breastfeeding—and bring your partner, too. These courses typically are offered through La Leche League International or local hospitals and can help you learn what to expect. They may even help you prevent common problems, such as engorgement. Once your baby is home, you might want to consider joining a breastfeeding-support group. These informal meetings are an excellent way to connect with other new mothers and share helpful tips and advice.

Every baby is different, but in general, a newborn up to about 3 months of age should nurse between 8 and 12 times a day.

3. "Room in" with your baby as much as you can

Having your baby stay in your room rather than in the hospital nursery is not only wonderful for your baby, it's great for you, too. "'Rooming in' allows you to learn your baby's feeding cues," says Wendy Haldeman, co-founder of The Pump Station, a breastfeeding-support center in Santa Monica, Calif. "It's a very important time to get to know one another." In addition, studies show that new moms actually sleep better when their babies are in the room with them.

4. Put your baby to your breast as soon as possible

Immediately after birth is the best time to introduce your newborn to your breasts. This is because babies have an alert phase that lasts for about an hour or two after they're born. "Newborns are primed for learning things at that point—that 'light bulb' is constantly going on," says Patty Janes, a lactation consultant and childbirth educator at St. Peter's University Hospital in New Brunswick, N.J. While your baby may not latch on and suck, he may start to lick or nuzzle you while you hold him close.

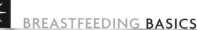
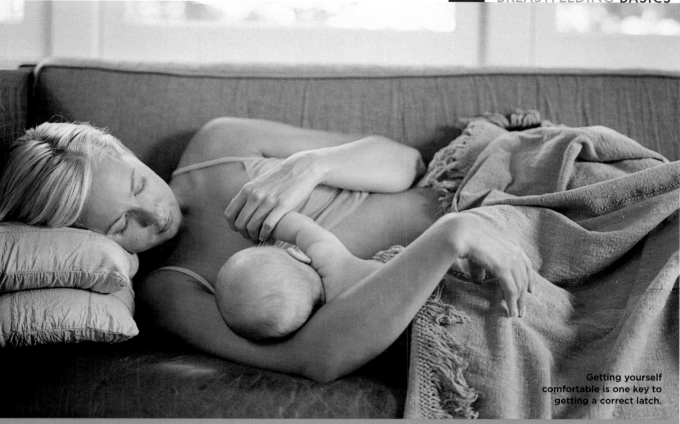

Getting yourself comfortable is one key to getting a correct latch.

5. Get the right latch

1. Position your baby on his side so he is directly facing you, with his belly touching yours. Next, prop up the baby with a pillow, if necessary, and hold him up to your breast; don't lean over toward him or stretch your breast out to him. (If you are lying down, tuck your arm underneath him.)
2. Place your thumb and fingers around your areola (the dark area surrounding your nipple).
3. Tilt your baby's head back slightly and tickle his lips with your nipple until he opens his mouth.
4. "Scoop" your breast into his mouth by placing his lower jaw on first, well behind the nipple.
5. Tilt his head forward, placing his upper jaw on the breast. Make sure he takes the entire nipple and at least 1½ inches of the areola in his mouth.

For a detailed guide, visit *www.fitpregnancy.com/breastfeeding*.

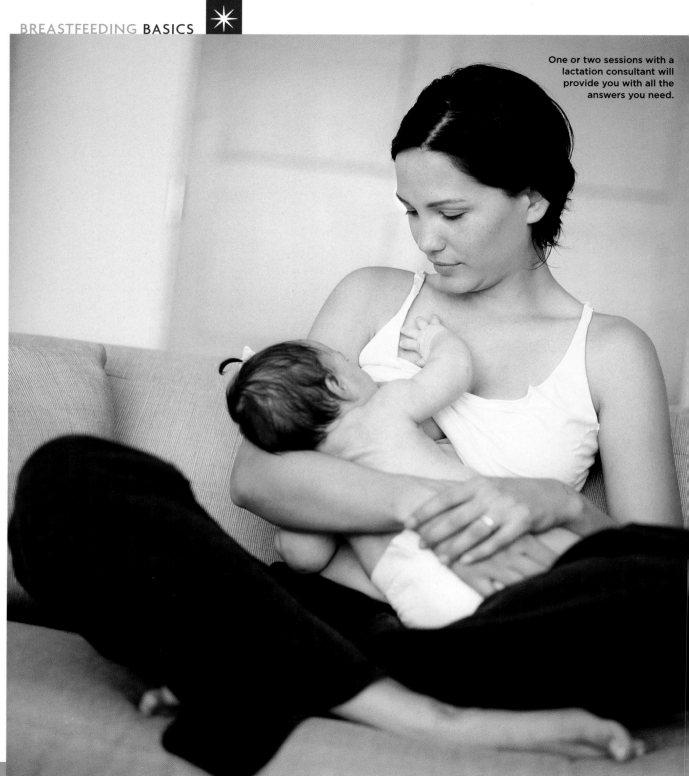

One or two sessions with a
lactation consultant will
provide you with all the
answers you need.

Some breastfed babies can sleep for about 6 hours by 3 months of age; others don't until 9 months.

6. Seek out support

If it takes a village to raise a child, then it's essential to set up a reliable support system when nursing. In fact, it's best to line up professional help while you're still pregnant. Some options:

> Lactation consultant Certified lactation consultants provide a wealth of support and practical information. Contact La Leche League International (*www.lalecheleague.org*), the International Lactation Consultant Association (*www.ilca.org*), Medela's Breastfeeding National Network (*www.medela.com*), your pediatrician or a local hospital to locate one near you.

> Pediatrician It's important to find a pediatrician who is supportive of breastfeeding. When you meet with a potential doctor, ask questions such as: How long should I exclusively breastfeed? If I'm having difficulties, what do you recommend? How long is breastfeeding beneficial? If you get a sense that the pediatrician is not pro-breastfeeding, keep looking.

> Friends and family "It's important to have someone who can tell you, 'Yes, I experienced that, too, and you'll get through it,' rather than having someone say, 'Are you sure the baby's getting enough to eat?'" Janes says.

7. Set small, realistic goals

It's wonderful to assume that you will breastfeed exclusively for six months, as the experts advise. But even the most committed nursing mother can encounter problems. And half a year may seem like an eternity if you end up with cracked nipples and engorgement (common consequences of not getting the proper latch). By breaking up that goal into shorter periods of time, you're more likely to hang in there even if you do encounter difficulties early on. Six weeks is a good starting goal.

8. Repeat after us: The laundry can wait

It's inevitable: A baby's arrival turns even the most well-run household upside down. Although it's easy to become overwhelmed by the dishes piling up, tell yourself that it's OK to let things go right now. Leave the chores to family or friends or hire a doula to help out. "All you should be doing those first few weeks is taking care of yourself and your baby," says Annette Leary, founder of Orlando Lactation and Childbirth Services in Orlando, Fla. On those days when you're feeling particularly beleaguered, remind yourself that housework and errands will always be there. But baby time, which seems so endless in those early, sleepless weeks, flies by in a heartbeat. Down the road, when you look back on these wondrous days with your baby, what you'll remember most is the magical time you spent bonding together—not whether you always put the laundry away.

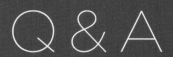

Q & A

>>> ANSWERS to your questions about breastfeeding your newborn.

Q Can I take a cold medication such as Claritin while I'm nursing?

A If possible, it's always best to avoid taking any type of medication while you're breastfeeding (and while you're pregnant). That said, if allergies, coughing or nasal congestion due to upper-respiratory infection are keeping you from sleeping, eating or participating fully in your (and your baby's) life, your doctor is likely to consider Claritin to help you cope with your symptoms.

Rest assured that after years of research on animals and humans, Claritin has been classified as safe to use during pregnancy and nursing. But even so, we think it is always best to use the minimum required dosage to achieve the relief you need.

Q I want to give my baby a pacifier, but I don't want to torpedo my breastfeeding. What's the real deal with nipple confusion?

A Early in the newborn period, the baby is learning how to breastfeed, and sucking from a plastic nipple—whether a pacifier or a bottle—is very different from sucking at the breast. It's therefore best to wait before giving your baby a pacifier or a bottle. "Babies don't come with labels that tell us which ones will be at risk for early weaning or breastfeeding problems if given an artificial nipple," says Nancy Erickson, R.N., I.B.C.L.C., a spokeswoman for the International Lactation Consultant Association. "That's why we say that it's better to wait to introduce a pacifier or bottle until a baby is 4 to 6 weeks old and is breastfeeding well."

Q Is it normal to feel pain during breastfeeding?

A "Some women do feel tenderness or discomfort when the baby latches on," says Corky Harvey, R.N., a lactation consultant and co-owner of The Pump Station, a breastfeeding-support center in Santa Monica, Calif. "But it shouldn't last for more than 20 seconds." Shooting pain, she adds, is a sign that something isn't right. If you experience such pain, it probably means that your baby isn't latched on properly and is sucking only on the nipple, rather than the nipple plus at least 1½ inches of the areola. (See tips on getting a good latch on page 123.)

Q When will my baby sleep through the night?

A Every baby is different. That said, some breastfed babies sleep through the night—meaning for about 6 hours—by 3 months of age; others don't until about 9 months. Until then, Margot Mann, I.B.C.L.C., director of the Riverdale Lactation Center in New York City, suggests sleeping with the baby and nursing from the side-lying position, which will allow you to fall back asleep while you breastfeed. If you take the proper precautions to protect your baby from suffocation (remove padding such as a feather bed or wool mattress pad, make sure your comforter doesn't cover the baby, don't push your bed against a wall, etc.), your baby can safely nurse while you sleep.

Q How do I know if my baby is getting enough milk?

A "Watch and listen to your baby's sucking and swallowing patterns," says Erickson. A baby who is getting enough milk takes long, drawing sucks, and her swallowing is audible. "The pattern should be rhythmic, with some pauses between sucking bursts," she adds. "When the baby isn't getting much milk, her sucks are short and choppy." Another way to gauge whether your baby's intake is adequate is to monitor her diapers: She should have at least six to eight wet diapers a day, with an average of two or more bowel movements.

Q How do I know whether my baby wants to nurse because she's hungry or she needs comforting?

A You may not know the difference, and it shouldn't matter. "Sucking is one of a newborn's highest needs," Harvey says. Furthermore, sucking for comfort rather than for hunger can actually help you succeed. "Sucking triggers milk production," she explains, "so during the early weeks and months, it's important to let your baby suckle as often as she wants." You may notice that your baby's nursing demands wax and wane. That's because when she's going through a growth spurt, she will need to nurse more often, which in turn increases your milk supply.

Q Do I need to change my diet while I'm breastfeeding?

A Follow the same basic guidelines and precautions that you did when you were pregnant. In other words, eat a healthy, well-rounded diet and drink plenty of fluids—at least eight 8-ounce glasses a day. You may discover that eating certain foods upsets your baby's tummy, but there is no evidence that you should make drastic changes. The Environmental Protection Agency does advise that nursing mothers not eat shark, tilefish, swordfish and king mackerel because these fish may contain dangerous levels of mercury. You can safely eat 12 ounces per week of other fish, such as wild salmon, and shellfish. (See "Fish Tales," page 62, for more information.)

Q How often should I be nursing my baby every day?

A Each baby is different, but in general, a newborn up to about 3 months of age should nurse between 8 and 12 times a day. But rather than keeping a tally or trying to get your baby on a schedule, the most important thing you can do is pay attention to signals and feed her whenever she seems hungry. "Babies give hunger cues, including rooting, opening the mouth, turning the head and making fussing noises," says Mann. "Crying is the cue of last resort."

Q If I give my baby an occasional bottle of formula, will she not want to breastfeed anymore?

A As long as you wait until your baby is about 6 weeks old, giving your baby formula occasionally probably won't affect her willingness to breastfeed or take breast milk from a bottle. But giving your baby bottles of pumped breast milk rather than formula will increase her ability to fight off certain diseases. "The baby's gut is an open structure, like a honeycomb, until about 5 months of age," Harvey explains. "Breast milk creates good bacteria that help close up the open walls of the intestines, in turn preventing the large molecules of some harmful bacteria and viruses from passing through."

Rather than trying to get your baby on a schedule, feed her whenever she's seems hungry.

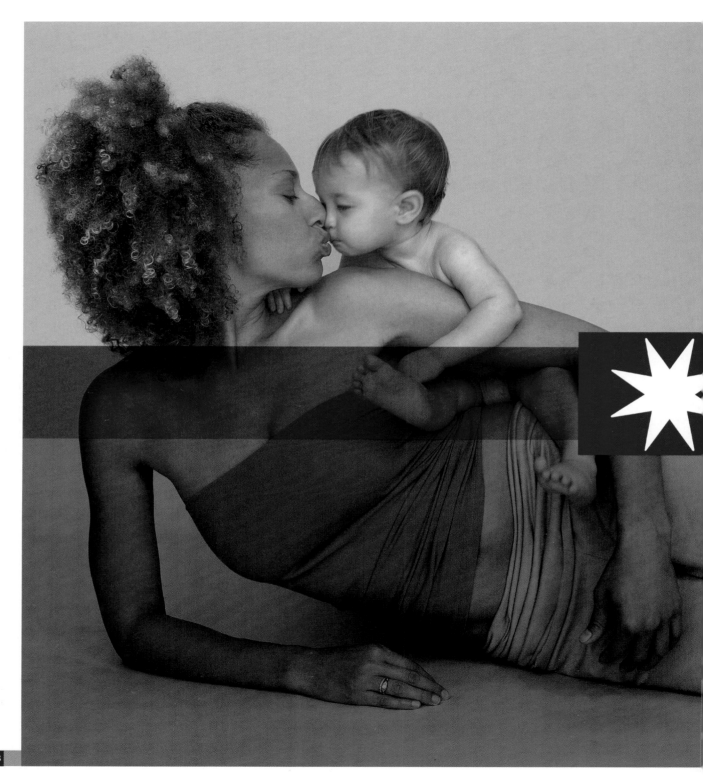

lose your baby weight

Shed pounds safely after giving birth—and get your body back!

>>> FROM THE MOMENT the pregnancy weight starts to accumulate, most women begin worrying about how to drop the pounds after their little one arrives. Once your baby is born and your days gradually regain something resembling a routine, it's time to turn your worry into action. If you're not sure how to begin, turn the page: We offer seven proven strategies (and four of the most effective toning exercises) for working your way back to your prepregnancy bod. Plus—since we know you'll be pressed for time—we've created three 10-minute postnatal workouts, all of which you can do with your new baby. Who knows? After following our advice and performing these workouts, you may be stronger and leaner than you were before you became pregnant!

in this chapter:
* 7 weight-loss tips
* 10-minute workouts you can do with your baby
* 4 great full-body moves
* your new body

7 weight-loss tips

>>> BREASTFEEDING, NAPPING, strength-training—all of these are tried-and-true methods that can help you lose your baby fat. According to research, new moms who participate in structured (i.e., weekly) postpartum diet-and-exercise programs are more successful at losing weight than moms who try to do it on their own (see No. 7 on page 135). If you decide to join a new-mothers' group, be sure to bring along this chapter. The other moms will definitely thank you!

1. get up and move

Most brand-new moms are too sleep-deprived and overwhelmed to even think about exercise. That's perfectly OK, says exercise physiologist and postpartum-fitness expert Renee M. Jeffreys, M.S., of Covington, Ky. Most women discover that their bodies aren't ready for serious exercise until six weeks after giving birth, anyway—longer if they've had a C-section.

Start by getting outside and taking an easy walk for a few minutes as soon as you feel up to it, Jeffreys says. If it feels good and doesn't cause or exacerbate bleeding, walk a little farther the next day. Do this until your six-week checkup, after which you should be ready to ease into 20 to 30 minutes of cardio exercise three to five times a week.

Grab your baby
and start moving.

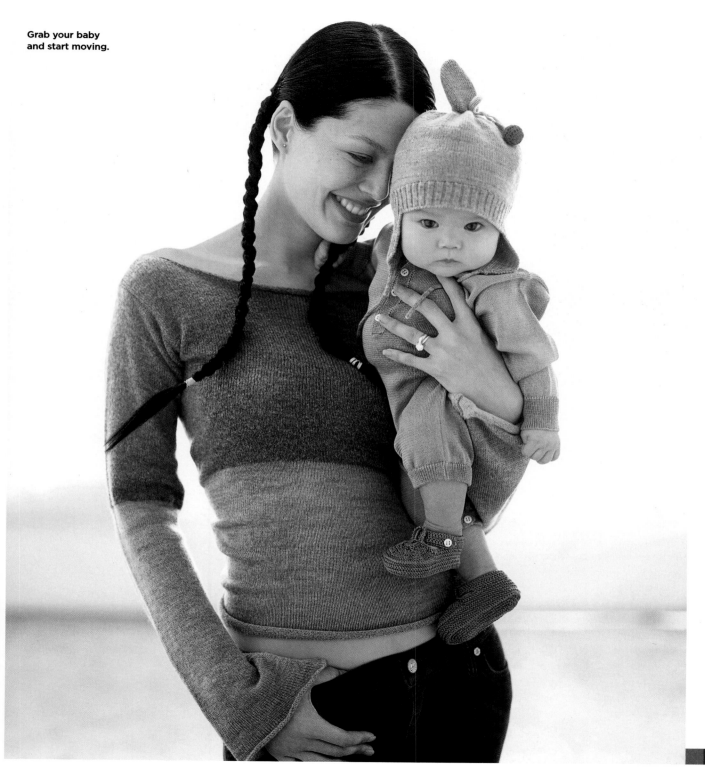

2. breastfeed

When you're breastfeeding, you'll probably need an extra 500 calories every day (that's about 2,700 total calories each day). And since nursing burns 600 to 800 calories a day, you still could be losing weight even if you can't find the time to exercise. Be aware, however, that as soon as you taper off or stop breastfeeding, or begin supplementing your baby's diet with solids, your calorie needs will plummet. You really could pack on the weight if you don't adjust your calorie intake downward and/or your exercise upward.

3. do resistance training

Resistance training is a great way to burn calories and regain your strength. At about six weeks postpartum and with your doctor's OK, invest in a set of 3- to 8-pound dumbbells and try to work in a postpartum weight-training video a few times a week; make sure it includes a warm-up and stretches. One of our favorite videos is *QuickFix Post Natal Workout* (visit *www.current wellness.com* to order), which features three 10-minute strength-training segments by fitness expert and mom Nancy Popp. You can also try our "Workouts For You and Baby" on page 136 for a fun way to strength train using the weight of your baby as resistance.

Get some more weight-bearing activity during strolls with the baby. Walk with him in a front carrier and you've got an all-natural 10- or 12-pound weight. Or push your baby in a stroller up hills to give your thighs and butt a fierce workout. (In addition, see our "Total-Body Strengtheners" on page 138.)

4. watch your calorie and fat intake

Say no to empty-calorie foods such as sodas, cookies, cakes and potato chips, as well as to fad diets that restrict entire food groups. Instead, eat a variety of nutrient-rich meals containing lean protein, whole grains, fresh fruits and vegetables and plenty of low-fat dairy products, says Tammy Baker, M.S., R.D., a Phoenix-based dietitian. And try to spread out all those fresh vittles. Consuming small, frequent meals throughout the day will keep your blood-sugar levels steady and help prevent overeating, Baker says. Keep in mind also that if your calories are distributed throughout the day, they're metabolized more efficiently and are less likely to be stored as fat. In addition, watch your juice intake—it's high in sugar and calories. All the vitamin C you need for one day is in a small glass of orange juice.

Nutrition experts advise against going on any kind of weight-loss diet right after giving birth. "To get your body back, you have to think about your health first," Baker says. "Your body is working to repair itself."

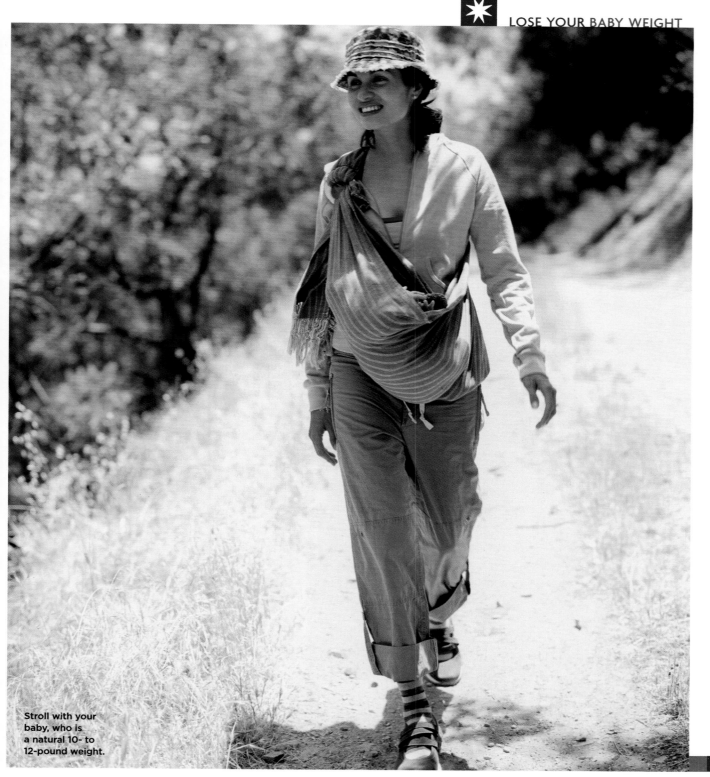

Stroll with your baby, who is a natural 10- to 12-pound weight.

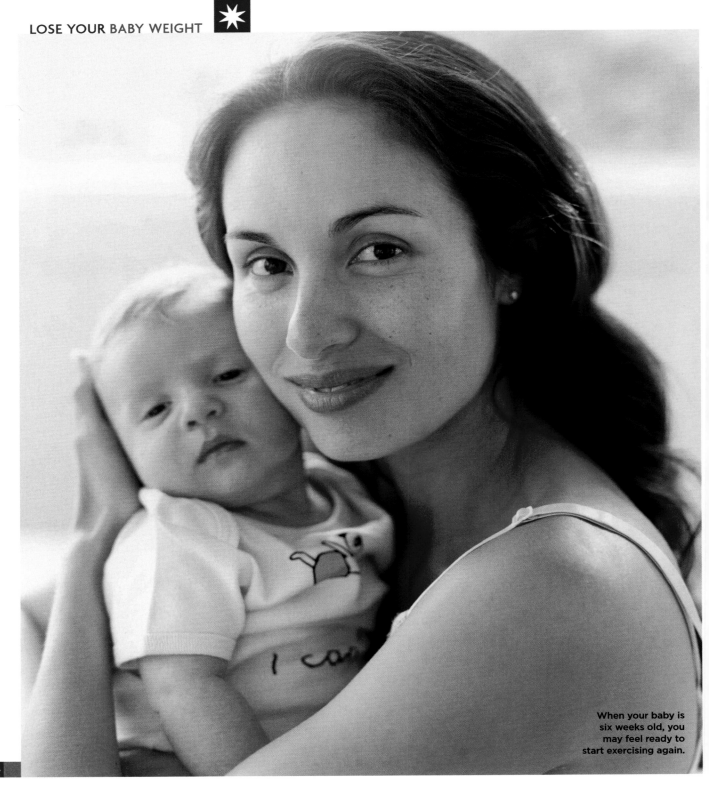

When your baby is six weeks old, you may feel ready to start exercising again.

5. take naps

"Getting plenty of sleep has been shown to help with weight loss because you're not compelled to binge on high-calorie, high-sugar foods for energy," says Sheah Rarback, M.S., R.D., director of nutrition at the Mailman Center for Child Development at the University of Miami School of Medicine. Strange sleep cycles like those forced on you by a newborn baby can upset your metabolism and make it more difficult for you to lose your pregnancy weight, Rarback says. Be sure to take a nap when the baby does if you need to—housework be damned. That way, you won't end up with a long-term sleep deficit, and you'll keep your energy levels—and food cravings—in check.

6. snack smart

Eating too many refined ("bad") carbohydrates can send your blood-sugar levels on a roller-coaster ride. And when your blood sugar drops, you're more likely to eat the first thing you can get your hands on. So skip the sugary and starchy treats. To avoid temptation, keep only nutritious foods at your fingertips. Stock up on low-fat milk, cheese and yogurt for snacks, as studies have shown that the calcium these foods contain can aid weight loss by preventing the hormonal response to store fat that's triggered by inadequate calcium. Also, eat high-fiber snacks such as figs, raisins, whole-wheat crackers and raw vegetables. They fill you up as well as help with digestion and regularity.

7. get with other new mothers

It can be helpful to connect with other moms for regular exercise. Example: When Carolyn Pione was a new mother in Cincinnati, she didn't feel she had the energy or the time to exercise after she had her baby. Then, some pals who had formed an early morning running group showed up on her doorstep urging her to join them. At first, Pione, who had gained 38 pounds during her pregnancy, couldn't keep up. But before long, she felt compelled to catch up, and besides, she didn't want to miss out on the friendly conversation. She lost all her baby weight and now runs in 5ks, something she never would have been able to do without the help of the group. "Alone, it would have been impossible," Pione says.

workouts for you and baby

>>> YOU DID IT: You made it through labor and delivery and you are now home with your new healthy baby. Your time is filled with breastfeeding, napping, diaper changing and cuddling as you care for this helpless new being.

But perhaps now more than ever, you need to take care of yourself, and exercise is an essential aspect of that. "Exercising either alone or with your baby can help you get your life back to normal after giving birth," says Gayle Peterson, Ph.D., a Berkeley, Calif., therapist who specializes in pregnancy and parenting. "Exercise not only helps you get your body back, but it also releases hormones that can help prevent the blues many new moms experience."

If you don't have the time or inclination for a long walk or formal workout, that's OK. Research has shown that several 10-minute spurts of exercise can be just as effective as one longer session. When you're feeling up to it and with your doctor's go-ahead, probably around six weeks postpartum, try these quickie 10-minute workouts. The goal is to do three quickies a day when you have the time, for a total of 30 minutes of exercise daily. So grab your baby and start moving. You'll both love it.

quickie no. 1: baby dancing

Dancing provides a light cardio workout involving all the major muscle groups. It improves balance and coordination and is a nice time to bond with your baby.

Select any kind of music that you enjoy and that makes you want to move. (Mix slow and fast songs for variety.) Hold your baby in your arms or use a secure front carrier. Keep a hand on the baby at all times and be sure to support your baby's neck. Move your feet, lift your legs and move your hips from side to side. Have fun, but avoid unnecessary bouncing or jarring movements. Remember to use your arms if your baby is in a carrier, reaching above your head and around you.

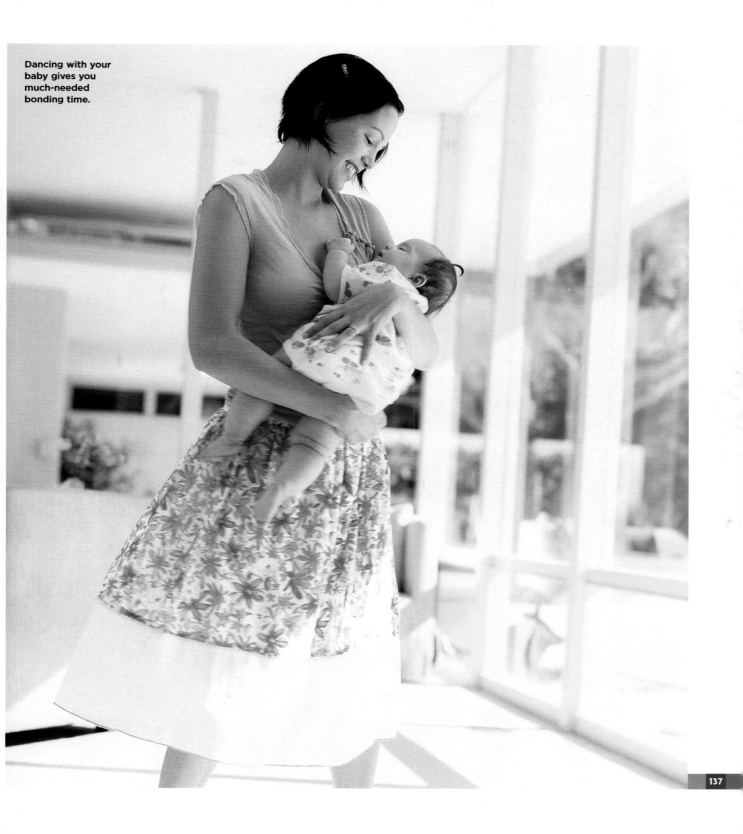

Dancing with your baby gives you much-needed bonding time.

quickie no. 2:
total-body strengtheners

Yes, you'll gain upper-body strength from carrying your new baby, but you also need to target your lower body and the muscles that were taxed during pregnancy and labor. The following four moves will help you build overall body strength.

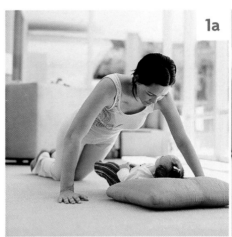
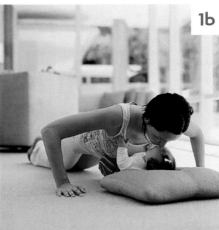
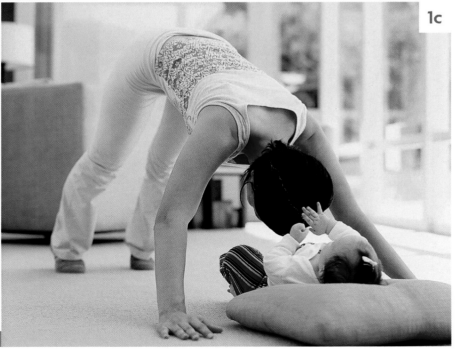

1. PUSH-UP KISS

Get down on your hands and knees. Place your baby faceup on a large pillow under your chest (A). With your knees behind your hips, wrists wider than shoulders, abs contracted and neck straight, bend your elbows to lower your chest toward your baby; kiss her (B). Slowly straighten arms and legs as you press hips toward ceiling to form an inverted V, heels approaching floor (C). Slowly lower back to starting position on knees. Repeat for 2 minutes, about 20–25 reps. *Strengthens chest, triceps and front shoulders; stretches hamstrings and calves.*

2. BABY ELEVATOR

Hold your baby securely, either face out or toward your chest. Stand with your feet wider than hip-width apart, knees slightly bent, abs tight (A). Bend your knees, bringing your thighs as close to parallel to the floor as possible, keeping knees behind toes (B). Rise slowly without locking knees. Repeat for 3 minutes, about 20–25 reps. *Strengthens quadriceps, hamstrings and buttocks.*

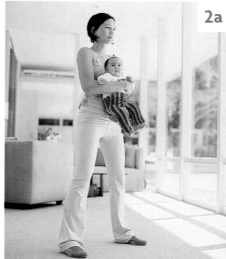

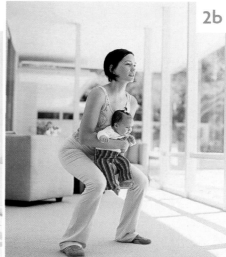

3. REVERSE-CURL PEEKABOO

Lie faceup and bring your knees toward your chest. Place your baby chest down on your shins (A). Holding her there, contract your abs to gently tilt your hips up off the floor as you lift your head, neck and shoulders to play peekaboo (B). Lower and repeat. Repeat for 2 minutes, about 20–25 reps. *Strengthens abdominals.*

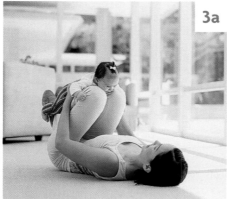

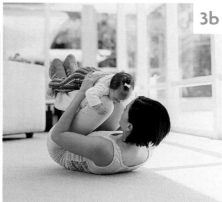

4. BABY BRIDGE

Lie faceup, knees bent, feet flat on floor and parallel, ankles under knees. Place your baby on your hips, just below your bellybutton, and hold her securely (A). Keeping your head on the floor, lift your hips to form one straight line from shoulders to knees. Pause at the top, squeezing buttocks and thighs, pressing into heels (B). Slowly lower to return to starting position. Repeat for 2 minutes, about 20–25 reps. *Strengthens thighs and buttocks.*

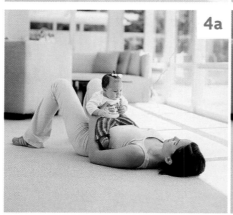

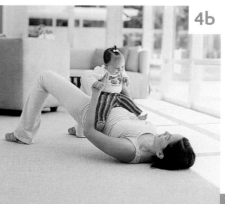

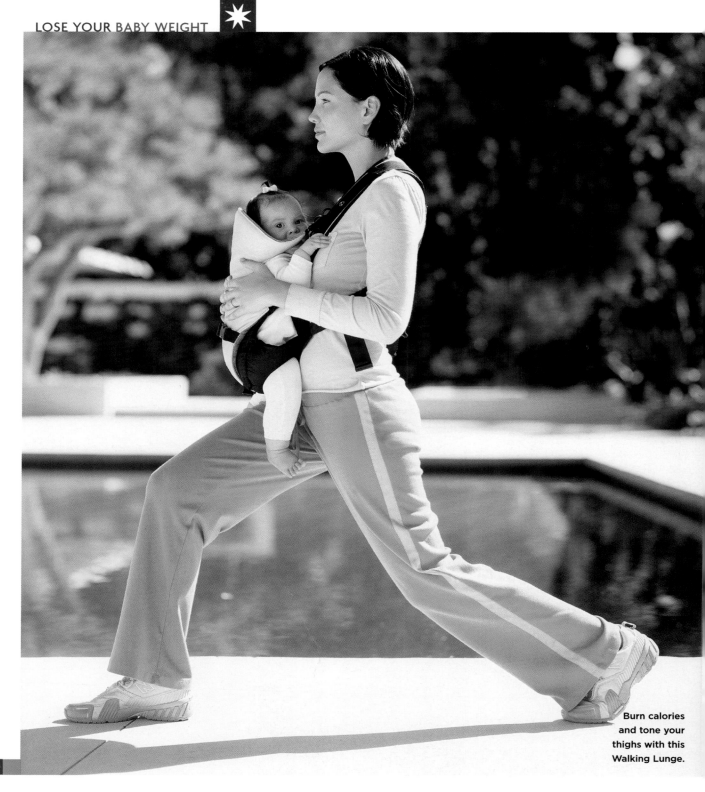

Burn calories
and tone your
thighs with this
Walking Lunge.

quickie no. 3:
walking and lunging

Walking and lunging combinations are an easy, effective way to blast calories, strengthen your heart and tone your quadriceps, hamstrings, buttocks and calves. Alternate 2 minutes of fast walking with 1 minute of lunges.

BRISK WALKING Place your baby in a secure front carrier. Before you begin walking, stand erect with your shoulders pulled back and down, abdominals drawn in. Pull your chin back so your ears line up with your shoulders. Breathe deeply, inhaling through your nose and exhaling through your mouth. Keep an eye on the path in front of you.

WALKING LUNGE Contract your abs and take a large step forward with your right foot, keeping your torso erect; do not lean forward or backward. Lower your torso and bend your knees until your right thigh is as close to parallel to the ground as possible and your left knee approaches the ground (shown, opposite). Push off your left foot to return to standing and repeat with the opposite leg. Keep your eyes level and watch the path in front of you.

If you eat 100 fewer calories every day, you could lose up to 10 pounds in one year. (Just don't try this while you're nursing.)

what is diastasis?

Diastasis is a separation of the outer rectus abdominis muscle that often occurs during pregnancy.

To check: Lie on your back with your knees bent and feet flat on the floor. Place your fingertips horizontally 2 inches above or below your navel. Exhale as you slowly lift just your head. Press gently and feel for a separation the width of three fingers or more, and a soft area in the midde—that's a diastasis. If you have one, try splinting when you do ab exercises or using a front carrier.

To splint: Take a strong piece of fabric that's about 62 inches long and 6 to 9 inches wide. Wrap it flat around your lower back, holding a section of the cloth in each hand (don't make a knot). Pull gently from both sides toward the middle over your bellybutton. If you had a C-section, wait until your incision has healed.

get your body back: 4 great moves

This workout will flatten your belly and make you strong all over. At about six weeks postpartum, after your doctor has cleared you of diastasis (see page 141), start with 8–10 repetitions, building up to 15. When you can complete 15 reps of all four exercises, add another set of 15 reps, resting 60 seconds between sets. To purchase an exercise ball, call Spri Products at (800) 222-7774 or visit *www.spriproducts.com*.

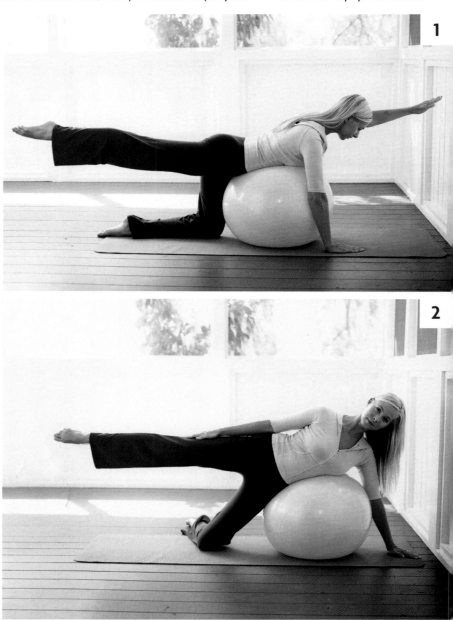

1

2

1. SUPERWOMAN

Kneel facing the ball and drape your torso over it. Place your hands shoulder-width apart on the floor in front of the ball, neck in line with hips. Inhale, then exhale as you extend your left arm in front of you and right leg behind you (shown). Hold for one full breath. Inhale and lower to the starting position, then exhale as you repeat with the other arm and leg (this is 1 rep). *Strengthens back, buttocks and shoulders.*

2. SIDE LEG LIFT

Draping your left side over the ball, put your left hand on the floor. Extend your right leg to the side, placing the foot lightly on floor, right hand on thigh, abs drawn in, shoulders relaxed. Keeping your hips and shoulders square, inhale, then exhale as you lift your right leg to hip height (shown). Hold for one full breath. Lower foot to floor, complete reps, then switch sides. *Strengthens upper hips.*

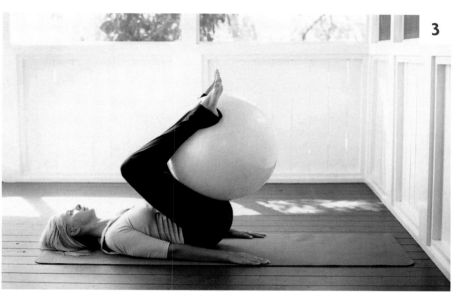

3

3. REVERSE CURL

Lie on your back with your legs farther than hip-width apart, gripping the ball with your legs. Arms are extended at your sides, palms down. Draw your abs in so your lower back is in contact with the floor. Inhale, then exhale as you use your abdominals to lift the ball, gripping it with your legs (shown). Slowly release the ball to the floor, keeping your abs drawn in and your lower back in contact with the floor. *Strengthens abs.*

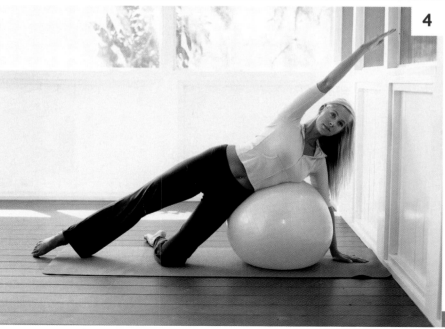

4

4. MERMAID ARC

Kneel on your left knee next to the ball and extend your right leg out, foot flat, left hand on the ball, right hand on right thigh. Inhale, and as you exhale, draw your abdominals in and lean your torso onto the ball. As you reach your left hand over the ball to touch the floor on the other side, reach your right arm up and over your body in an arc (shown). Hold for one full breath. Inhale and return to starting position, complete reps on this side and then switch. *Strengthens and stretches the entire torso.*

your new body
(what stays, what goes)

Here's what's in store for your body during the first year after having a baby:

Within two weeks Don't be surprised if you still look about five months pregnant. Let's say you gained 30 pregnancy pounds. During delivery, you immediately lose about 15 pounds, leaving up to 15 more that will take time to burn off. Also, your uterus has been stretched to 25 times its normal size—you'll have a floppy pouch where your baby used to be. As your breasts produce milk, they also add a couple more pounds.

At six weeks Your uterus should be back to its original size, and a few more pounds of water weight will be gone. Your doctor probably will give you the green light to resume exercising.

Within one year As long as you've been active and eating sensibly, you can expect to be back to your original weight, though it may have shifted. The size and shape of your breasts may be permanently changed, your hips may be wider and there may be little pockets of fat in places where there weren't before. But it's not the size of your bluejeans that matters—it's how healthy and fit you are!

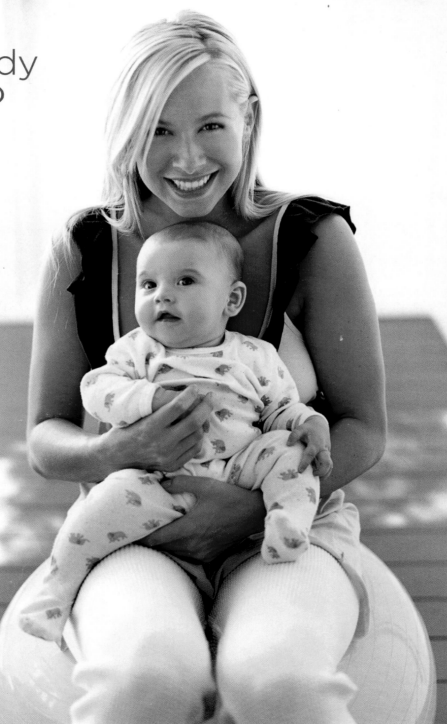